Recent Research in Psychology
Applied Behavioral Science

JON F. MERZ

Louis A. Morris

Communicating Therapeutic Risks

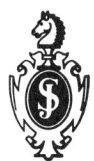

Springer-Verlag
New York Berlin Heidelberg
London Paris Tokyo Hong Kong

Louis A. Morris
The American University, Food and Drug Administration
Gaithersburg, Maryland 20877, USA

Library of Congress Cataloging-in-Publication Data
Morris, Louis A.
　　Communicating therapeutic risks.
　(Recent research in psychology. Applied behavioral
　science)
　Includes bibliographical references (p.　　)
　1. Communication in medicine.　2. Therapeutics—Complications and sequelae.　I. Title.　II. Series.
R118.M65　1990　　　615.5′07　　　　89-26141

Printed on acid-free paper.

©1990 Springer-Verlag New York Inc.
All rights reserved. This work may not be translated or copied in whole or in part without the written permission of the publisher (Springer-Verlag New York, Inc., 175 Fifth Avenue, New York, NY 10010, USA), except for brief excerpts in connection with reviews or scholarly analysis. Use in connection with any form of information storage and retrieval, electronic adaptation, computer software, or by similar or dissimilar methodology now known or hereafter developed is forbidden.
The use of general descriptive names, trade names, trademarks, etc., in this publication, even if the former are not especially identified, is not to be taken as a sign that such names, as understood by the Trade Marks and Merchandise Act, may accordingly be used freely by anyone.

Camera-ready copy prepared by the author.
Printed and bound by Edwards Bros., Inc., Ann Arbor, Michigan.
Printed in the United States of America.

9　8　7　6　5　4　3　2　1

ISBN 0-387-97192-0 Springer-Verlag New York Berlin Heidelberg
ISBN 3-540-97192-0 Springer-Verlag Berlin Heidelberg New York

For my girls
Terry, Kate, and Jodie

Author's Note

I would like to thank the many colleagues who helped formulate the ideas expressed in this book and provided encouragement for writing the text. First, I would thank David Brinberg who offered me the opportunity to express my thoughts about risk communication in a coherent text, provided steadfast encouragement, and helped me communicate in a clear(er) voice.

I would also like to thank my colleagues at the Food and Drug Administration for their insight and support. Ellen Tabak's work on physician-patient communication and question-asking has provided intellectual linkages between the health education and cognitive psychology literatures. Her help in copy editing the book was invaluable. Nancy Ostrove deserves much credit for ideas about emotional coping. She has done much to move my thinking away from pure cognitive rationalizing.

The encouragement of Michael Mazis at The American University has been exceptional. Mike consistently challenges his colleagues to bring out their best. His willingness and ability to devote his time and energy to inspire and support intellectual achievement is remarkable. Stimulating discussions with Jack Swasy have helped me think through many complex issues and find consistent themes in a morass of conflicting theories.

Finally, I would like to thank David McCallum and Sharon Hammond at Georgetown University Medical Center. They have broadened my views and helped me to conceptualize this work as part of the emerging field of risk communication.

The views expressed are solely those of the author. This book was written in my capacity as a private citizen. No official support or endorsement of the Federal Food and Drug Administration or The American University is intended or should be inferred.

Louis A. Morris
Food and Drug Administration
and
The American University
September, 1989

Contents

Author's Note vii

1. Introduction 1
2. Learning About Therapy 9
       Why Communicate Risks? - The Health
           Professional Perspective 11
           Barriers to risk dissemination 12
       Why Communicate Risks? - The Patient
           Perspective 13
           Patient preferences 13
       Motivation to Seek Risk Information 15
           Medical decision making 16
           Coping with threats 17
           Avoiding risk Information 20
       The Content of Risk Communication 22
           Risk communication stages 23
       Sources of Risk Information 25
           Patient preferences 25
           Sources utilized 26
           Segmentation pattern 27
           Risk seeking passivity 28
       Stimulating Risk Disclosure 30
           Question-asking studies 31
           Increasing patient involvement 34
       Implications 37

3. Physician's Risk Disclosure 39
Normative Studies of Doctor-Patient Communication 40
Observational analyses 40
Patient interviews 41
Information Exchange Standards 43
Risk Disclosure Factors 45
Physician's script 46
Moderating Factors - The Physician 47
Individual differences 47
Role and attitude 49
Moderating Factors - The Prescribing Environment 52
Disease and treatment 52
Patient perception 55
Situational factors 59
Implications 60

4. Patient Information Processing 63
Attention to Risk Information 64
Priming effects 64
Comprehension 68
Context-availability model 69
Integration in Memory 72
Schema 72
Categorical schema 72
Ad hoc schema 74
Scripts 76
Elaboration 76
Processing Risk Communications 79
Information Retrieval 81
Retrieving evaluations 82
Implications 83

5. Patients' Medical Judgments 85
The Patient as a Decision Maker 85
Decision Making Processes 87

                Editing stage 88
                Evaluation stage 89
        Biases in Decision Making 90
                Framing effects 90
                Interpretation bias 91
                Recall biases 92
                Weighing and evaluation bias 93
                Motivation to make decisions 94
        Patient Consent and Risk Acceptance 96
                Patients' role 96
                Optimal decision making 97
                Physician and patient perspective 98
                Assessing probabilities 99
                Risk perception 100
        Risk Communication and Compliance 102
                Reasons underlying noncompliance 103
                Limiting treatment 104
        Implications 107

6. Effects of Risk Communication 109
        The Initial Doctor Visit 111
                Expectations and outcomes 112
                Emotional reactions 113
                Need fulfillment 115
                Initial therapy evaluation ... 115
        Product Use 116
                Suggestion induced side effects 117
                Product misuse 120
        Treatment Evaluation 120
                Product liability 122
                Medical malpractice 124
        Maintaining Treatment 127
        Implications 131

7. Mass Media Risk Communication 133
        Historical Development of PPIs 134
                Phase one - the flirtation ... 134

    Phase two - infatuation 135
    Phase three - the "break-up" 138
    Phase four - the maturing
           relationship 139
  Assessment of PPI Effects 142
    Patient knowledge 143
    Regimen adherence 145
    Doctor-patient relationship 146
    Returned prescriptions 146
    Conclusion 147
  Direct Advertising of Prescription Drugs 147
    Manufacturer rationale 148
    Risk disclosure requirements 148
    Political environment 150
    Survey data 151
    Sales experience 151
  Risk Disclosure in Television and Magazines 152
    Purpose of risk disclosure 152
    FDA study 153
    Knowledge results 154
    Attitude results 155
    Conclusion 155
  Implications 156
    Endnote 157

References 159

1
Introduction

I guess everyone has a cousin Ernest. He is the fellow of whom your mother asks..."Why can't you be more like your cousin Ernest?" Cousin Ernest went to the high school for genius children and got all A's, even in French. As the years went by, I lost contact with Cousin Ernest. Then last year, at a family gathering, I met him again. Sure enough, he had gone to Harvard and become a doctor, a radiologist.

We began discussing his practice and he mentioned that he performs some fairly risky diagnostic tests. While legally he was compelled to tell patients about the risks they were undertaking, he said that risk disclosure was a useless exercise. "No one has ever refused to undergo the procedure," he said.

It was difficult to argue with his observation that no patient ever refused to undergo his tests. I understood that the lack of refusals did not necessarily mean that risk disclosure was a useless exercise, but his underlying argument was quite compelling. If patients did not use risk information to make a decision about treatment, was the disclosure of risk information useful? Was risk disclosure simply a legal protection exercise, performed for the doctor's benefit rather than the patient's? Why should a health professional disclose risks if patients do not use the information to evaluate a test or treatment and make a personal judgment about their willingness to undergo the procedure?

I had worked on the issue of risk disclosure for pharmaceuticals for some time and had consulted on informed consent topics. There was a large literature supporting the patient's desire to know about the risks of treatment and there were numerous ethical arguments justifying the importance of equalizing the relationship between the doctor and patient. There was also some research on the routine disclosure of risk information when treatments were prescribed or administered. However, most of this research was philosophical or descriptive. There was little research to explain why patients did, or did not, want to know about the risks of treatment. There were few models to explain the conditions under which health professionals disclosed risks or patients asked questions. There was precious little discussion of what patients did with the risk information that they received.

As I read more about these topics, I learned that useful models did exist in related literatures that might explain why patients did, or did not, want to know about the risks of treatment. There was also a growing body of research on how risk information is cognitively processed and used by patients. Lastly, there were also some interesting technological and political initiatives on the horizon that might dictate how the risks of pharmaceuticals may be communicated in the future.

Thus, cousin Ernest continues to influence my research. This book seeks to address his concerns: what is the value of communicating therapeutic risks to patients, to what extent do people obtain therapeutic risk information, and how is it used? The book is divided into six chapters that intertwine descriptive research from the health communications literature with informational processing and emotional coping literatures.

The *second chapter* addresses the basic question of why patients want to know about the risks of treatment. Our hypothesis is that risk information seeking is a form of anticipatory coping. Seeking risk information is a logical method of appraising and responding to the threats and uncertainties posed by significant life events. We generally conceive of coping as a response to illness rather than its treatment. However, the threats posed to a patient occur in stages. When first diagnosed, we view therapy as a means of coping with illness. Over time, however, toxicities and side effects of treatment pose significant threats to health and safety. Learning about the risks of treatment is necessary to understand, control, and hopefully master the threatening therapeutic environment. The "two edged sword of medicine" makes therapy both a "means" and a "cause" of coping with threats.

Of course not all patients seek risk information. Some may be unaware that therapies pose risks and others may avoid risk information as a means of coping with its threats. Segmenting patients according to risk information seeking patterns helps us understand how risk information is differentially sought by various groups of patients. When this segmentational study is done, however, we see an overwhelming passivity of patients when obtaining therapeutic advice. While some of the passivity is motivated by avoidance coping, a great deal more appears due to lack of knowledge and skills at asking health professionals for the information. Recent research on patient activation suggests that patients can be taught to actively question health professionals to obtain the information they need about the risks of treatment.

The *third chapter* focuses on the doctor as the individual most in control of risk disclosure. The medical sociology literature highlights many obstacles to therapeutic risk communication. What therapeutic advice do doctors routinely convey and what factors influence disclosure patterns? When patients are asked about routine therapy they report being told remarkably little about its risks. However, when physicians report what they tell patients about therapy, a considerable amount of risk information is cited. This "Grand Canyon size gap" between doctor and patient report is more than a simple problem of patients' forgetting some details of the interaction. The measurement of risk communication must focus on the very basics of how physicians phrase risk disclosures and how patients interpret their advice. For common therapies, physicians communicate using a habitual disclosure pattern or "script." The "script" is "written" to minimize patient management problems and to avoid raising fears that the physician cannot easily dissuade. Thus, the risks of using a medicine are not mentioned directly. Rather, the information is phrased as precautions for the patient to take or directions to avoid further harm. For example, patients may be told to avoid driving when taking a drug that makes them drowsy. For most conventional therapies, unavoidable risks are not routinely incorporated in the "script" that physicians use to guide their conversation. This chapter focuses on the factors that influence the development and execution of the physician's "script." How do individual doctors adapt their therapeutic disclosures to fit their patients' needs, their own proclivities, and the pressures of the immediate environment?

Even if informed, patients may have great difficulty understanding risks and placing them in perspective. The *fourth chapter* switches focus from the doctor to the patient. The patient is perceived as a processor of risk information. The cognitive psychology and consumer behavior literature suggests that people have severe limitations on their ability to select, comprehend, integrate, evaluate, and retrieve communications. What factors influence whether patients pay attention to risk disclosures? Unfortunately, the logical ordering of risk disclosures during the course of the doctor visit works against effective communication. The placement of therapeutic risk information at the end of the visit corresponds with attention deficits to the latter parts of the therapeutic interview. "Priming" patients either before or during the interview to pay attention to therapeutic risks can increase the communication of that information. Simply placing risk information at the beginning of the interview also increases its communication. Unfortunately, effective communication involves a series of trade-offs. Increased attention to risk information decreases attention to other aspects of the interview.

Even if patients attend to risk information, the meaning ascribed to the communication is problematic. Medical conversation is often criticized for its use of jargon. Complicated medical terminology can be unintelligible. It can also be quite educational, giving patients vivid and memorable keystones for organizing the torrent of new information that they must assimilate. Making medical words meaningful tools that add perspective rather than obstacles to circumvent is an important goal for professional-patient communication. Understanding how the patient makes sense of medical terminology points to the importance of the "context" of the communication, rather than the words themselves, that help people understand important messages.

For medical information to be useful it must be stored in memory in a way that serves the patient's needs. Our memory system is highly organized based on how we think we will use important information. The organizing framework or "schema" used to store risk information determines how we integrate this information in memory. We gain perspectives on therapeutic risks by associating those risks with other concepts stored in memory. Risk information may be "categorized" with other therapeutic effects, "scripted" into an expected action sequence, or organized on an "ad hoc" basis when unique needs arise.

Finally, how we store information in memory determines the meaning we secure when the information is retrieved. Risk information should help us form an evaluation of a treatment. If we have already formed an evaluation, we can retrieve it if the treatment is reapplied. If we have had little experience with a treatment, the best we can do is retrieve the most relevant information in memory and "construct" an evaluation based upon what we know. When explicit information is lacking (such as personal experience with the treatment), situational influences (such as our view of the treating doctor, our relationship with the institution, and momentary discomfort) has a larger role influencing therapeutic evaluation.

An evaluation permits us to form some judgment about the treatment we are undertaking. The *fifth chapter* considers three results of the therapeutic evaluation process: choice, consent, and compliance.

We consider the use of therapeutic risk information to enable patients to make a *choice* about their treatment. Cousin Ernest's perspective is clearly limited to his field of practice. Patients are often faced with dilemmas that require them to make a choice about undergoing or selecting treatment. Prospect theory helps us organize the patient's decision making processes. Two stages are postulated where patients initially "edit" relevant evaluative criteria and performance levels for different therapies. Secondly, they "evaluate" options based upon a systematic review of the alternatives or some heuristic short-cut. Biases in the editing and evaluation phases can prejudice the decision and decrease the patient's autonomy and control over selecting desired treatments.

The *informed consent* literature often equates patient consent to treatment with decision making. Our view is that consent is a passive process in which risk information is shared with the patients.

Once risk information is disclosed and understood, the patient may rationally refuse treatment. However, as cousin Ernest observed, this is a rarity. Rather, consent permits the patient the autonomy to cope with known risks in a fashion that befits the patient. The patient may actively seek additional information, seek social support, intellectualize the threat, deny the possibility of a serious threat, or engage in some other coping strategy.

How the patient perceives the treatment (primary risk appraisal) determines the nature and extent of coping (secondary risk appraisal). The risk perception literature suggests that patients do not evaluate therapeutic risks on the basis of their pure probability and severity of outcomes. Other factors that personalize the risk are taken into account when risks are appraised. Two important risk evaluation elements are the "dreadedness" of the outcome and the "control" that the patient exercises over the threatening event. Thus, permanent paralysis is more dreaded than death, and the risk of a fatal accident that can be potentially prevented by the patient's actions is viewed as less upsetting than the risk of a tumor that is beyond the patient's control.

The final section of the chapter focuses on behavioral consequences of risk communication. For the health professional, providing risk information can be an effective persuasive device to foster *medically compliant* behavior. In a rational world, patients are motivated to achieve a positive health status and avoid illness. However, good health is but one of many competing goals. Momentary incentives and distractions may diminish longer term goals. For example, sailors taking hypertensive medication have been known to avoid taking their drugs (which reduce sexual ability) on the days when the ship is in port.

Certain therapies can be dangerous if overused and health professionals may need to detail the risks of prolonged treatment to frighten patients not to use more than the prescribed amount. However, fear appeals have limited, short-term effects on health behavior. The conditions under which risk communication will be effective are highly restricted. It is important for health professionals to understand the motivational properties and limits of fear appeals in influencing behavioral change.

The *sixth chapter* concentrates on the outcome of risk communication. If patients are informed about the risks of treatment, along with its benefits, are they more satisfied with their care? Studies of patient preferences indicate that more complete communication is one of the most desired elements for improving patient care. However, prospective research suggests that fuller communication does little to improve satisfaction ratings. It is apparent that risk communication, although desired, is unexpected. It is the patient's expectation and view of how physicians commonly behave that determines satisfaction. Thus, greater risk communication may do little to improve satisfaction ratings.

On the other hand, if a patient experiences an adverse effect and is not preinformed of its possibility, the patient may become angry and upset. A trust has been violated. Norm theory suggests that the perception that it is "easy" for doctors to tell patients about the risks of treatment amplify emotional reactions.

Thus, there is good practice management rationale for physicians to inform patients about therapeutic risks. Unfortunately, many physicians believe that preinforming patients about the risks of treatment increases the likelihood that adverse effects will occur because of suggestion. Empirical research has disabused this myth. Informing patients about side effects does not increase the number of side effects patients report. It does, however, increase the attribution of experienced bodily state changes to the side effect action of the administered drug, which may have both benefits and dangers for the patient.

A final consequence of informing patients about therapeutic risks is its influence on later treatment evaluations and legal action. Both product and malpractice liability cases have been decided on the basis of risk information provided prior to treatment. Furthermore, some legal opinion extols that suits may be averted in the first place if patients are preinformed about risk possibilities and given the option of refusing treatment.

The *seventh chapter* switches focus from interpersonal to mass media communication. In recent years we have seen a greater amount of therapeutic risk communication through both print and electronic media. Two case histories are presented. The first case discussed is government's requirement for written leaflets or *patient package inserts* (PPIs) to accompany the distribution of prescription drugs. In the United States there have been four phases in the development of PPI policy, starting with their requirement for a few selected drugs, moving to plans for larger scale implementation, a total withdrawal of the program, and progressing back to their requirement for a few selected drugs. In Europe, the direction of PPI policy has taken a different course. By 1992, with the advent of the European Economic Community, PPIs will be required for most prescription medicines.

In addition to an historical review of PPI development, research evaluating PPI effects is also critiqued. Generally, PPIs have been shown to increase knowledge about the less commonly known facts about prescription medication, especially the risks of treatment. However, their influence on behavior, either positive or negative, appears to be quite limited to short term, easily influenced actions.

The second case discussed is the development of *direct to consumer advertising* of prescription drugs (DTCA). A limited number of manufacturers have expressed an interest in advertising their products directly to consumers. FDA risk disclosure requirements make it necessary to incorporate product risk information within the advertisements. Results are presented from an FDA study of television commercials in which differing contents and formats for product risks were studied. We conclude that vivid and distinct risk disclosures are necessary for patients to discern and remember the risk information. As with physician provided instructions, vivid risks may detract from communication of product benefits. Therefore, concerns about public health protection and commercial freedom of speech must be carefully weighted in the development of public policy in this area.

2
Learning About Therapy

Modern medicine has blessed us with a number of highly effective treatments. We can control, cure, prevent, or alleviate a wide variety of conditions and diseases. Infectious diseases that were once the major cause of mortality have been controlled or eradicated by vaccines and antibiotic drugs. We can treat myocardial blockages with surgery and replace worn out or broken body parts with human or mechanical ones. Specific and useful therapies have been developed for cardiovascular disease, cancer, diabetes, arthritis, ulcers, and many neurological and psychological problems.

There is much in the therapeutic armamentarium to generate hope for the modern patient. Unfortunately, there is also much to generate fear. Modern therapeutics carries a great cost, not only in a financial sense, but in a physical sense as well. Although medical treatments have become more specific and powerful, they all work by altering the structure and function of the human body. The biological and physical mechanisms for modern medical treatment have remained essentially the same as in prescientific days; they cut, burn, and poison. Although we hope to "cut, burn, and poison" selectively, the treatments we administer are powerful and their adverse consequences can be both profound and severe.

Risk/benefit decisions are implicit in any therapeutic choice. We assume that the benefits of a treatment have been assessed, compared to its risks, and that a therapy is administered only when its benefits outweigh its risks. Treatment restrictions and licensure exams ensure that only individuals with sufficient training and expertise make these risk/benefit decisions. Except for over-the-counter medication and home remedies, patients do not routinely select their own treatment. Valid information about the risks of treatment is essential for the health professional making treatment decisions.

But what about the patient? Should we communicate information about therapeutic risks to people undergoing treatment? Do patients want to know about the risks of treatment? Don't patients put themselves in the hands of doctors precisely so they won't have to worry about treatment risks? Is there any reason why patients should know about treatment risks? Over the past decade we have learned the answer to these questions: *patients need and want to know about the risks of treatment.* However, their desire is often left unfulfilled because they don't know that this information exists or they are unwilling or unable to obtain the information.

In this chapter we will first examine why patients need to know about the risks of treatment. From the health professional's perspective, societal pressures stemming from technological innovations in treatment, a more sophisticated patient-base, and ethical concerns about patient autonomy have fostered increased risk communication. However, barriers to effective risk communication still inhibit health professionals from informing patients about treatment risks.

Notwithstanding these societal pressures, patients themselves overwhelmingly signify a desire to know about the risks of treatment. The reason for this desire to know is not immediately apparent. To some extent it is based upon the wish to participate more fully in the decision to undergo treatment. Our premise, however, is that risk information seeking is also a coping response. Knowledge of treatment risks provides patients the opportunity to physically and emotionally prepare for the negative outcomes of their treatment, gaining mastery and control over their environment.

The second part of this chapter focuses upon the process of communicating risks. What risk information do patients need and how do they obtain the information? When patients are first diagnosed and coping with initial notification that they have a serious disease, information about therapeutic risks is unimportant and may be counter-therapeutic. Later, as patients progress through this initial phase and begin to cope with their "career" of taking treatments, therapeutic risk information becomes more important. The ongoing relationship with a health care provider who supplies risk information when it is needed and desired by patients is a comforting and satisfying alliance.

The physician provides the bulk of therapeutic risk information. However, other health professionals also provide risk information, as do non-professional friends and relatives and non-personal sources such as books, manuals, and mass media. Of course, not all patients want to know about therapeutic risks or have the skills to actively seek it out. A certain segment of the population neither obtains risk information nor shows any desire to pursue it. Even those patients who say they receive risk information display an overwhelming passivity in its receipt, idly waiting for the physician to provide the information without asking any questions.

How can we stimulate patients to obtain more information? In recent years there has been a fascinating line of research indicating that under certain conditions, patients can be activated to ask questions. How can we motivate and educate patients to learn more about their treatment? Modern health care requires activated patients, to actively administer treatments and to actively learn about the risks they undertake.

Why Communicate Risks? - The Health Professional Perspective

Over the past decade, it has become evident that patients need to (1) become more aware of treatment procedures, (2) understand the risks posed by the therapy, and (3) become involved with administering and monitoring their treatment. Only with increased involvement can we expect patients to benefit from administered care and avoid complications of unsuccessful therapy or its adverse consequences. There are three societal trends that provide concurrent rationales fostering greater therapeutic risk communication: patient education, medicolegal concerns, and medical marketing.

First, the *patient education* movement has fostered greater risk communication. Alarmingly high numbers of patients fail to follow directions for administering their own therapy. Between 30% and 50% of patients significantly deviate from prescribed therapeutic regimens, jeopardizing the success of their treatment. At least part of the failure to follow prescribed regimens can be traced to inadequate communication of therapeutic information to patients (Morris and Halperin, 1979). Patients cannot administer and monitor their treatment if they do not know what to do.

Thorough communication of risk information is important so that patients can (1) avoid contraindicated behaviors, (2) obtain early treatment for serious but unavoidable side effects, and (3) monitor bodily state changes for signs of toxicity. The need for greater patient education about therapy is increasing, as the population ages and requires more complex treatment regimens, as therapies become more advanced, as cost controls favor greater home care, and as patients take more responsibility for their own health care.

Secondly, the *medicolegal movement* has increased the flow of risk information to patients. Fully informing patients about the risks they face when undergoing therapies has become essential to fulfill the patients' legal right-to-know. Unless patients are fully informed about a treatment's risks and, at least implicitly, consent to undertaking those risks, health care providers increase their liability if adverse effects do occur. The prospect of legal challenges to the physician's practice of medicine has fostered greater risk communication and record keeping to assure that the patient's consent to treatment can be documented.

Thirdly, the pressure on doctors to more aggressively *market medical care* has increased the flow of benefit and risk information to patients. It has become a sign of good practice management to more fully inform patients about their therapy. Better communication not only serves the patient's cognitive needs, but it serves emotional needs as well. Patients may prefer doctors who spend more time explaining treatment to them. As medicine becomes more competitive and "consumer-driven," physicians are becoming more responsive to the patient's desire for health information.

Barriers to risk dissemination

Although the patient education, medicolegal, and marketing in medicine movements all present strong reasons for better risk communication, there are also strong reasons inhibiting risk communication. Health care providers often view the prospect of providing negative information to patients as fraught with obstructions and uncertainties (c.f., Taylor and Kelner, 1987). For example, in a survey of 501 primary care physicians, a majority of respondents said that suggestion induced side effects and patient resistance of drug therapy occurred occasionally in their practice and 12% to 19% said these problems occurred frequently (Boyle, 1983). In comparison, only one-fourth of the sample said that serious adverse drug effects occurred occasionally in their practice and only one percent said that they occurred frequently.

In addition, most of the physicians surveyed (79%) said they spent about the right amount of time informing their patients about therapy (4% said they spent too much time and 16% too little time). Time pressures and practice demands were cited as the major barrier by those who said they spent too little time informing patients about treatment.

Why Communicate Risks? - The Patient Perspective

Although the three movements fostering risk communication are surely having an effect on the practice of medicine and the communication of therapeutic risks, it is unclear how fully these trends have penetrated the practice of medicine at the level of a single doctor conversing with a single patient.

In the medical marketplace, it ultimately will be the patient that determines the value of risk information. If patients need and want this information, then health care providers will begin to disseminate it. Understanding patient preferences regarding risk communication furnishes an initial glance at the demand function that will drive risk communication activities.

Patient preferences

Surveys that have directly measured patients' preferences about health information invariably find that the majority of patients state they want to know more about their treatment, especially the risks of treatment. In a survey conducted by the CBS Television

Network (1984), subjects were asked to rate the value of 27 categories of information related to drug therapy (e.g., directions for use, cost, methods of administration, contraindications, side effects). Over half of the subjects rated each of the 27 information categories as highly important. The side effects of prescribed drugs, however, was rated as the single most important piece of information that people wanted to know about their medication.

Subjects in the CBS study also rated how well informed they were on each of the 27 information categories. Perceived knowledge about drug effects varied with the category. The relative "knowledge gap" could be identified for each of the categories by comparing the "importance" and "well informed" ratings. On average, the knowledge gaps for safety and efficacy categories were greater than for the other categories. The "mean knowledge gap" was 50% on drug the safety and efficacy categories (approximately 27% of the sample believed they were well informed about safety and efficacy whereas 77% believed that it was very important to learn about these issues). The "mean knowledge gap" on proper usage categories was 30% (50% of the sample believed they were well informed and 80% believed that it was important to learn about these issues). The authors of the study concluded that information about the safety and effectiveness of treatment was the largest informational need expressed by patients.

The amount of risk information desired by patients appears to be greater than generally divulged by doctors or other health professionals. Faden, Becker, Lewis, Freeman and Faden (1981) asked patients and parents of pediatric patients to signify which of 16 risks and 5 benefits of Dilantin (a neurological drug) they would want to be informed about prior to consenting to treatment. More than 90% of both samples selected every benefit and over 80% of both samples chose all but two of the risks. In contrast, the majority of physicians surveyed reported that they routinely informed patients of five or fewer of the 16 risks.

In a study conducted for the President's Commission for the Study of Ethics in Medicine and Biomedical and Behavioral Research (Abram, 1982), members of the general public and physicians were queried about the disclosure of treatment risks. Both doctors and the public agreed that patients should be informed about side effects that were likely to occur, with physicians somewhat more assertive than the public that expected or common risks should be divulged. Eighty-five percent of the public believed that physicians should initiate discussion of common risks and 95% of the physicians stated that they generally do. Only 13% of the public and 2% of physicians felt that patients should ask for information about common risks.

This tendency toward physician assertiveness was also apparent for the disclosure of risks of a 1/100 chance of serious disability; 75% of the public believed that physicians should initiate discussion and 81% of physicians stated that they generally do. About 22% of the public and 16% of physicians believed that patients should ask for this information.

However, as the probability of treatment risks decreased, there was greater disagreement about risk disclosure. Physicians became more reserved about risk communication while patients retained their desire for risk information. Two-thirds of the public (64%) believed that physicians should inform patients about a 1/1,000 chance of serious disability or death compared to half (52%) of the physician sample. One-third of the public (33%) and 40% of the physicians felt that patients should ask for this information.

Many doctors apparently believe that only patients who want information about serious but rare therapeutic risks should receive it. Question-asking is the signal that patients want to know about these risks. Physicians may not realize the barriers patients face asking for this information.

Motivation to Seek Risk Information

Clearly, patients want to know about therapeutic risks, even risks with extremely rare possibilities. It is reasonable that if patients are aware of early warning signs of a side effect, they can take protective action. However, in many cases, serious but rarely occurring risks are unavoidable. In spite of what patients say, does providing such information help patients? Giving patients this information forces them to confront frightening and uncontrollable events that are highly unlikely.

The health professional is faced with a dilemma. Why terrorize patients unnecessarily when the fear could be easily avoided by simply not disclosing the information? In some cases the health professional does not have a choice. Risk information must be provided. Medicolegal considerations have institutionalized risk disclosures for serious but unavoidable risks for certain medical tests and procedures. For most medical treatments, however, informed consent procedures are not required. Physicians have the discretion to disclose, or not disclose, what they view as medically necessary. As we shall see in the next chapter, given this option, patients are often uninformed about unavoidable risks, or informed in a way that disguises the risky nature of the treatment.

Medical decision making

Why then give patients information about the risks of treatment? The most frequently cited rationale for informing patients is increasing their role in medical decision making. Only if fully aware of the risks and benefits of treatment can patients determine which risks they are willing to face. If fully informed about the risks and benefits of treatment, the patient can govern, or at least participate in, the therapeutic decision making process. Medical malpractice cases have been determined on the basis that the patient would have selected to avoid treatment if the risks of treatment were more fully communicated.

Although greater participation by patients in medical decision making is the most often cited reason why patients want to know more about the risks of treatment, it is not the only reason underlying the desire to learn about treatment risks. Furthermore, medical decision making may not be the most compelling reason for communicating therapeutic risks to patients.

Berwick and Weinstein (1985) examined the value that patients place on medical information. From the patient's perspective, 44% of the value of obtaining an additional medical test pertained to uses of the information outside of the medical decision making context. For example, information about the risks of treatment might change the way patients plot their own life course or how they evaluate different elements in their life.

In a study by Strull, Lo and Charles (1984), patients and physicians were asked to signify or estimate patient preferences for information and decision making in hypertension therapy. Compared to patients' stated preferences, physicians were more likely to underestimate than overestimate patients' preferences for information about therapy. However, physicians tended to overestimate rather than underestimate patients' desire to participate in making decisions about treatment.

Furthermore, patients are unlikely to countermand or disagree with their physician's advice when choosing a therapy. In a study by Povar, Mantell and Morris (1984), patients underestimated the role that the physician's advice had in influencing their beliefs about the acceptability of different remedies. Although patients were notably risk averse in their decision to undergo different treatments, the provision of risk information did not negatively influence the decision to undergo therapy if the physician had endorsed the treatment.

Coping with threats

If patient decision making is not the reason why patients desire to know about the risks of treatment, why then would patients want to know about unavoidable therapeutic risks? Research on how patients adapt to the threat of illness elucidates why risk information serves the patient even if it is not used to make a therapeutic choice.

When people first perceive physical symptoms, they must appraise why the symptom occurred to understand how to react. Whether or not the patient seeks medical care is a function of several factors. Not only must the patient perceive the symptom as a sign of illness, but the patient must believe that professional care is needed and that the benefits of care outweigh its costs (Safer, Tharps, Jackson and Leventhal, 1979). Although the degree to which symptoms are disruptive, threatening, and painful are the major factors determining the extent to which symptoms are perceived as a sign of illness, the degree to which the patient is familiar or uncertain about the symptomatology is most predictive of seeking professional advice (Jones, Wiese, Moore and Haley, 1981).

Thus, for the patient who enters therapy, not only is there physical disruption, there is also a great deal of uncertainty about the illness and the therapy. Information provided by the physician may help the patient adjust to the threat posed by the illness. The biological course of the illness is only one of several threats. Patients need to know more than just the physical course of the illness to fully adjust to the threat and disruption. Different types of information are necessary to psychologically adjust to the illness and its treatment.

Taylor (1983) has suggested three themes that underlie patients' cognitive adaption to threatening events such as the initial experience of symptoms or the diagnosis of a serious disease. First, the patient seeks to understand the meaning of the experience in an attributional sense. Information about the cause and course of the illness may help the patient appraise the experienced symptoms. By understanding the cause of the event patients may answer nagging questions about why their illness occurred to them. The search for meaning also allows patients to rethink attitudes and priorities so they can get on with their life's work.

Secondly, patients seek to regain mastery and control over the threatening events and their own lives. When ill, the patient's traditional role is one of a passive recipient of care. External events, such as the illness, and other people, such as health care providers, control how patients are to behave rather than patients themselves. While disease information may help patients understand why they became ill, information about administered treatment helps assure that patients can control adverse consequences of therapy.

Rothbaum, Weisz and Snyder (1982) have proposed if people cannot change the environment by making it conform to their own wishes (primary control) they may bring themselves into line with environmental forces (secondary control). They propose four ways in which secondary control can operate. First, merely being able to predict the course of treatment may prevent the violation of expectations and severe disappointment. Secondly, control may operate in an illusory fashion. Although the likelihood of an event occurring may be due to chance (outside of the patient's ability to control its outcome), some individuals believe themselves to be "lucky" or "unlucky," attributing greater control to how they perceive the environment habitually treats them than objective reality dictates. Thirdly, patients may attribute greater control of treatment outcome to the physician. By aligning and identifying themselves with this powerful individual, patients may exercise control vicariously. Fourthly, all of these attributions provide patients with greater ability to interpret the meaning of otherwise uncontrollable events and accept their occurrence.

The third theme of Taylor's cognitive adaption model is that patients seek to enhance their own self-image and esteem. Patients may engage in behaviors that make them feel better about coping with their illness. Not only can risk information reduce uncertainty about additional negative occurrences but by becoming knowledgeable about the treatment patients may feel more self-assured and confident about their own ability to take care of themselves. As postulated above, even if self-deceptive, just being able to interpret the meaning of events makes people feel better about themselves.

One of the notable findings from the President's Bioethics Commission study was that physicians base their willingness to disclose risks on the likelihood that the risks will occur. Probability of occurrence is not a significant factor determining the public's desire to know about therapeutic risks. People signify a desire to know about even extremely low probability events.

Why is the public less sensitive to risk probabilities than health professionals? It is often hypothesized that the public does not understand probabilistic information and, therefore, disregards it. However, if patients utilize risk information for coping purposes rather than decision making, probabilistic information may not be as valuable for patients as it is for health professionals.

When formulating decisions about which treatments to select, the likelihood of serious risks is a major factor to consider, especially when choosing among options with variable benefits and risks. For coping purposes, risk probability is less important. Patients have great difficulty translating public health probabilities to make predictions on an individual basis. A 1/100,000 probability of disability translates to a 0 or 1 outcome for the individual patient (either the patient becomes disabled or does not). If patients perceive a threat, they are motivated to cope with it. In the next section we will examine some of the coping mechanisms that patients use to adjust to and control the threats posed by their treatments.

Avoiding risk information

Although most patients want to know about the risks of treatment, some patients prefer not to obtain risk information. There are several reasons why these patients do not desire additional risk information, some of which are motivational and others of which reflect communication difficulties.

Weinstein (1988) has suggested a stage model that helps explain how beliefs about risk communications interact and influence behavioral responses. First, patients must be aware that a hazard exists for them to initiate some behavioral change. Secondly, they must believe that the risk is significant and worthy of their attention. Thirdly, they must believe that they themselves are vulnerable to being harmed by the risk object or event.

During the course of an illness patients may be differentially distributed along each of the stages of Weinstein's model. Many patients may be unaware of the risks of treatment, especially if they are unfamiliar with the therapy. Patients may not consider that treatments that are apparently unobtrusive, such as radiation, ultrasound, or acne medication, could have dangerous side effects. Even if aware, patients may not believe that the risks caused by the therapy are serious. For example, parents may not understand that childhood diarrhea, a side effect of many pediatric antibiotics, can be an extremely serious problem. Finally, with the extremely low probabilities of many serious side effects, patients may not believe that they are vulnerable to the adverse effects of treatment, especially if they are otherwise active and healthy. Some patients may cognitively reinterpret extremely low probability risks as zero personal probability in order to simplify and understand information about the therapy. Research on risk interpretation following genetic counseling sessions indicates that parents interpret small absolute percentage chances of birth defects as "lower level" risks than do health professionals providing the information (Wertz, Sorenson and Heeren, 1986).

Risk avoidance may also be a motivated coping response to a threatening environment. Using Taylor's framework, we may view risk information processing as a form of anticipatory coping with threatening events. Two basic forms of anticipatory coping are possible, vigilant and avoidant (Kiyak, Vitaliano and Crinean, 1988). Vigilant coping takes the form of seeking information about the risks of therapy and avoidant coping takes the form of not seeking this information. Although it was originally presumed that vigilant coping was superior to avoidant coping (Janis and Mann, 1977), more recent reviews find little systematic superiority of one form of coping over another. Suls and Fletcher (1985) suggest that avoidant coping may have superior short run benefits and vigilant coping may be superior in the long run.

In a broad review of coping strategies, Roth and Cohen (1986) also concluded that coping styles may be summarized on the basis of whether the patient avoids or approaches (attends) threatening stimuli. The authors suggest that there are costs as well as benefits to adopting different coping strategies. For the patients who use an approach strategy, there may be increased distress and nonproductive worry. However, these patients may be able to take appropriate action, resolve the trauma they face dealing with the realities of their illness and its treatment, and emotionally ventilate using appropriate avenues. For patients using an avoidance strategy, there may be a lack of information that prohibits them from making optimal decisions about how they can best adapt to their treatment. However, these individuals may increase secondary control, as they may attribute greater control to their physician or utilize mechanisms such as prayer that permit them to accept their lack of control over the situation.

We postulate that individual preferences for risk information are a strong determinant of post-event outcomes. Consistency of the risk communication with preferred coping style may facilitate adjustment. Unfortunately, coping styles may change over time. As a disease may run an unstable course, so may an individual's informational needs and coping styles.

The Content of Risk Communication

Whether or not risk information helps patients adjust to threatening events depends on the hierarchy of immediate and long term goals the individual is attempting to achieve at any point in time. Taylor (1983) contends that information, and the cognitions that result from the information, are not robust elements that maintain their meaning across situations. Rather they are "strategic changing elements that serve general value-laden themes." As a patient's goals change, risk information may be helpful, irrelevant, or disruptive. The value of obtaining specific categories of risk information will vary over time, across individuals with different information seeking proclivities, by virtue of providers' information dissemination patterns, and will depend on the consistency of the information with the patients' existing state of knowledge.

Motivational changes during the course of treatment direct the particular type of risk information that patients find meaningful. At different times, patients' and doctors' views fluctuate about the important elements of therapeutic information exchange. As the patient progresses through "patienthood," certain types of risk information become relevant as other elements become irrelevant.

For example, when first becoming ill, the immediate need to understand and adjust to the illness dominates the patient's goals. Information about the risks of treatment are of little value for this purpose. As the patient adjusts to the illness, needs for mastery and self-enhancement become more important and risk information may help attain these goals. In addition, risk information may be valuable, useless, or disruptive depending on how the information is presented in comparison with the patient's cognitive structure and immediate goals. For example, information about unavoidable side effects (e.g., "there is a 1 in 10,000 chance that the therapy causes blood dyscrasia") without providing information about how to cope with side effects if they occur, may frustrate an individual trying to actively master a threatening environment. However, a physician may present additional information that helps the patient achieve mastery goals (e.g., "blood dyscrasia can be treated with additional medication so we will have to take monthly blood tests to see if they occur").

The data on patient preferences may be interpreted as indicating that patients generally view risk information as helping them to achieve coping goals. At certain points in time, certain patients may avoid information that frustrates attempts to achieve these goals. Some patients may prefer to avoid risk information totally as a general adaptation strategy. Other patients may take more situationally driven perspectives on risk information seeking. If information is presented at an appropriate time, in a supportive and personally meaningful fashion, a risk information avoider may become a risk information seeker. Therefore, to understand risk information seeking patterns, it is important to understand general risk information seeking proclivities as well as situational factors that moderate the desire for risk information.

Risk communication stages

We can organize the elements of a risk communication strategy by reference to stages in therapeutic decision making. McCallum (1989) has identified three decision making stages through which an individual passes during an illness. Receptivity and desire for risk information are dependent on the patient's stage in this process.

The first stage is the "pre-decision" stage. No therapy has been prescribed and the patient may not even be diagnosed as ill. Risk information seeking may be determined by long term personal interest or "personal involvement." Certain individuals may have a long standing interest in health issues, new therapies, and the risks of treatment. These information seekers may be more likely to read newspaper and magazine articles about health innovations. If an individual has a long standing health problem, or a close friend or relative has such a problem, then that individual may focus on health seeking for treatments related to that illness. Learning as much as possible about these treatments (including the risks of treatment) would be a priority for these individuals. Limits on time, restricted access to information sources, lack of expertise, and the pressure of other priorities delimits general health information seeking proclivities.

The second stage is the "decision making" stage. During this period, the individual has been diagnosed and therapeutic options are considered. The diagnosis is usually made by a doctor or by patients themselves for minor illnesses. In this stage, the individual is most likely to actively seek out and consider information about the risks and benefits of possible treatments. To a great extent the doctor controls what risk information is disclosed during this period. Institutional informed consent procedures are likely only for the most serious or acutely risky treatments. The degree to which patients "participate" in the decision to undertake a treatment influences risk communication. The manner in which risk information is disclosed also determines the success of the communication. Doctors may fail to disclose therapeutic risks or disclose them in a fashion that does not successfully communicate their meaning or relevance.

The third stage of risk communication is the "post-decision" stage. Once a treatment has been chosen, the patient must follow prescribed dietary, behavioral, and medication taking regimens to avoid contraindications and assure that the treatment works as intended. Information about what precautions to take when undergoing therapy is important during this stage. Unfortunately, communication of therapeutic advice is difficult and patients often report poor knowledge of appropriate actions to assure maximum safety of the regimen. Other times, appropriate therapeutic advice is not disclosed. The patient's role as an active participant in health care is an important factor during this stage. The patient's role is not one of a decision maker, but as a monitor and evaluator of health outcomes. The patient must be aware of problems that necessitate a change in therapy and report these problems to the physician if they occur. Thus, long term relationships with health care providers become important.

For certain treatments, such as radiation therapy or some pharmaceuticals, risks increase as the treatment continues. Coping with long term accrued threats is particularly difficult. As the patient becomes more accustomed to the treatment, and perceives its benefits more fully, threats continue to grow. Rather than becoming more accustomed to the threat of the treatment, the patient may become more uncomfortable with it, forcing vigilant coping the longer the treatment continues.

Clearly, the particular type of risk information that physicians disclose and that patients seek depends on the stage in the risk communication process and the perceptions of the doctor and patient during this process. A physician may perceive that information about rare but serious unavoidable risks is important during decision-making but extraneous during the post-decision stage. Some patients, however, view risk information as important during all the stages because of the need to develop effective coping strategies as well as participate in the decision making process. Other patients wish to avoid risk information during all the stages because they do not actively seek to participate in therapeutic selection and view risk avoidance as a more adaptive personal coping strategy. How much and what type of risk information patients desire must be analyzed by taking into account not only individual differences in patients and providers, but where in the process of risk communication the patient is psychologically located.

Sources of Risk Information

Thus far we have considered only the physician as a source of risk information. During the past decade there has been an enormous growth in the number of health information sources available for consumers. While physicians remain the primary source of therapeutic advice, there are many other personal and interpersonal sources of health information. What is the role of each of these sources in communicating the risks, benefits, directions for using therapies? Research on the availability and use of prescription drug information provides a broad indication of source utilization.

Patient preferences

Polling data confirm that there is widespread acceptance of several different sources of prescription drug information. In a recent Harris poll (Baker, 1985), 88% rated the physician as a very important source of health information. However, the majority of respondents

(56%) also viewed the pharmacist and voluntary health organizations (53%) as very important sources. About one-fourth viewed friends and neighbors (21%) and government publications (27%) as very important. In a survey conducted by the Columbia Broadcasting System (CBS, 1983), most respondents rated the physician (95%) and pharmacist (84%) as useful sources of prescription drug information, but other sources such as mass media (33%) and family and friends (25%) were also rated as useful by some people. In a survey of people over age 45 conducted by the American Association of Retired Persons (Peguet, Wegner and Brown, 1984), most subjects rated the physician as an important source (52%) but also cited to a variable extent sources such as the pharmacist (25%), books (19%), newspapers (15%), magazines (12%), and television (11%) as important sources of prescription drug information.

All three surveys confirm the physician as the most important source of drug information. However, the pharmacist is also valued quite positively in all surveys. Nonprofessional and written sources of information appear somewhat acceptable, although to a much more variable degree.

This general pattern of information seeking was also found in a study of information seeking during pregnancy (Aaronson, Mural and Pfoutz, 1988). Health care providers were most preferred, followed by books, with media, family, and friends rounding out the list. In addition, women also cited themselves as a source of information, especially if they had a previous pregnancy. This suggests that internal (i.e., memory based) sources of information may be difficult for patients to use because of their lack of familiarity with the treatments. External sources of information must be viewed as the primary anticipated method of patient education for newly introduced therapies.

Sources utilized

Although surveys of patient attitudes indicate a broad acceptance of drug information sources, examination of the sources patients say they actually use and the type of information patients state they obtain indicate that risk information is frequently left uncommunicated. In a survey of 1,104 patients who had obtained new prescriptions during the previous month (Morris, Grossman, Barkdoll, Gordon and Soviero, 1984), 70% said they received some information at the doctor's office, mostly from the doctor (95%), and additionally from the nurse (12%). A little over half (about 60%) said they received directions for use information and about one-third (30%) mentioned refill instructions. Precautionary information was said to be delivered at about the same rate as refill instructions (32%) and information about side effects at a somewhat lesser rate (26%).

Recollections of verbal counseling at the pharmacy indicated considerably less information dissemination as approximately one-third said they received directions for use instructions, 16% precautions, and 11% side effect information. Structural barriers at the pharmacy were a notable moderator of pharmacy counseling. A little over half (58%) of the sample said they were handed the medication by the pharmacist, and counseling rates were two to three times higher when the medication was provided by the pharmacist rather than a cashier or clerk. However, written information was more likely to be provided at the pharmacy. A good proportion of the sample (70%) said they received informational stickers on the medication vial and 16% said they received a brochure, pamphlet, or instruction sheet. Only 5% said they obtained any written information about the medicine at the physician's office.

In addition to the doctor and pharmacist, 18% of the sample said they relied on their friends, relatives and neighbors. Drug reference books were cited by 16% of the sample, with 7% stating that they looked up their prescription in the **Physicians' Desk Reference** and 5% stating that they used a large variety of other consumer and professional reference sources. Magazines (6%), newspapers (4%), television (4%), and radio (1%) were cited infrequently as sources of prescription drug information. More technologically advanced forms of drug information (audio and video tapes, computers, etc.) were cited to a negligible extent.

Segmentation pattern

Normative descriptions provide a broad overview but they tend to treat patients in a uniform way and fail to account for differences in information seeking proclivities. To examine differences in drug information seeking patterns, Morris, Grossman, Barkdoll and Gordon (1987) utilized a segmentational analysis to sort patients into homogeneous, yet distinct, groupings. A four cluster solution appeared to best represent the data.

The physician reliant group (40%) was most likely to obtain direct counseling initiated by the physician and sought additional information as a reinforcement of the physician's directions. The pharmacist reliant group (19%) was the youngest segment. They were likely to obtain prescriptions for family members (often children) and tended to frequent independent pharmacies where they were more likely to interact directly with a pharmacist. The questioners (7%) were more likely to receive multiple prescriptions and perceived many barriers to obtaining information from health professionals. They were most likely to actively solicit information and consult reference books for information about the medication. The uninformed group (34%) was the oldest group and were least likely to receive any written or verbal information from health professionals. They were most likely to agree with the attitude statement that, "one need not ask questions if one trusts the doctor."

The segmentational analysis confirms different patterns of drug information dissemination for different patients. The size of the segments indicates that the majority of those obtaining any drug information rely on the physician as the main source and seek additional information to reinforce and augment the physician's advice. The large "uninformed" group also confirms that there is a sizeable group of people who do not receive, and see little need to obtain, drug information. This group may be composed of different subgroups that are at various stages in interpreting the threats posed by the treatment or may actively avoid risk information as a motivated coping strategy.

Risk seeking passivity

The data from these information seeking studies indicate an immense passivity on the part of patients to receiving therapeutic risk information. The relatively small size of the "questioners" segment suggests that few patients actively initiate conversations about therapeutic risks. Even for patients who receive information from the doctor or pharmacist there were few signs of active information search. Counseling tends to be delivered spontaneously by the doctor as only two to three percent of the respondents said they obtained information about any of the categories queried as the result of a question.

The lack of active solicitation of therapeutic risks is consistent with other studies that indicate that when patients do question the physician, the question tends to focus on nonmedical matters (Bain, 1979). Interestingly, when patients in the Morris et al. (1984) study had a question about the medication (especially about precautions or side effects) they were more likely to ask someone other than the doctor. This confirms anecdotal evidence that patients may not want to "bother" the doctor with a question about the adverse consequences of a medicine and are more likely to approach a more accessible staff member.

The lack of active solicitation of prescription drug information is consistent with the consumer behavior literature that identifies surprisingly little information search, even for high involvement items. Generally, information search is perceived as a costly endeavor. We have already seen that health professionals cite several barriers to providing risk information. Patients also perceive many barriers based either on the physician's behavior or on structural elements of the environment or the relationship (Morris, Grossman, Barkdoll and Gordon, 1987). These barriers may be translated to "cost factors" that patients (who know that the information exists) must be willing or able to overcome to obtain the information they want about the risks of therapy.

One important limitation of the Morris et al. (1987) survey must be noted. The survey's results reflect interactions only at the first appointment where medication was prescribed. As discussed earlier, patients' coping strategy may favor concentrating on understanding the cause and effects of the illness at initial doctor visits.

Interest in the therapy may develop later, based upon the patient's experience with the medication and adjustment to the regimen. However, additional studies suggest that questions about the risks of treatment are not increased significantly at later visits, unless there is a clear "trigger event" that stimulates the patient to take the initiative. Studying communications about prescribed medicines, Boreham and Gibson (1978) found that at the initial patient interview doctors provided information about the name, purpose, desired effects, and instructions for use to about one-fifth to one-third of patients. Information about adverse side effects was more likely to be delivered at revisits (to 15% of patients) when initiated by a patient's question. Most side effect questions were prompted by the patient's experience of the side effect.

Unfortunately, if patients' experience of an adverse drug effect initiates the active solicitation and subsequent communication of risk information, we are resolved to a Catch-22 situation. If a side effect is not experienced, the patient cannot know that the treatment poses risks. If adverse effects do occur, coping responses could not be planned because the patient is not told ahead of time. Thus, patients are not upset prematurely with frightening risk information. Nor, however, are they prepared to cope with adverse side effects if they occur.

Stimulating Risk Disclosure:

The realization that risk communication in the doctor-patient interview is limited has led to a number of initiatives to improve the flow of information between doctor and patient or to supplement the interaction with additional information. The National Council of Patient Information and Education (NCPIE) has initiated a national campaign to increase question-asking when medication is prescribed by doctors (Bullman and Rowland, 1986). In addition, a number of studies have examined methods to understand and increase question asking behavior.

Miyake and Norman (1979) studied question asking behavior among students taking a computer course. They found an inverted U-shaped relationship between question asking and expertise. Students who were novices were unable to form appropriate questions. They did not understand basic computer concepts and had no basis for understanding what information they lacked. Trained subjects asked few questions because they already knew the answers. In their study, question asking behavior rose when the level of complexity of the material presented matched the knowledge level of the audience.

The Miyake and Norman study suggests that patients may not ask questions because they do not have enough basic knowledge about therapy to know "what they don't know." In a more precise study of people's ability to assess their own knowledge about a domain, Glenberg, Sanocki, Epstein and Morris (1987) studied the "calibration" of comprehension. They found that the correlation between subjective assessment of knowledge gained from reading material and performance on an objective test was close to zero. The authors concluded that people assess personal knowledge about a topic by assessing their familiarity with the general domain rather than on what they have learned from a particular source of information. Thus, if patients believe they are somewhat familiar with a treatment from a previous medical encounter or from what they had previously seen or heard, they may not understand how little they know about the treatment. Patients who are somewhat familiar may believe that they are sufficiently knowledgeable about a treatment and have little need to learn more.

Providing patients with sufficient background may help them formulate questions about treatment. Several programs have been initiated that utilize retired health professionals to lecture elderly patients about general background principles related to medication taking and pharmacology. However, the technological complexity of the information and uncertainties about how the information is applied raises questions about the value of such programs. Although general primers about therapeutic safety may help, there have not been any evaluations to determine if general education increases question asking.

Question-asking studies

Rather than provide general education, a number of interventions have been tested that: (1) provide patients with specific questions they should ask, and (2) motivate question generation in clinical practice. To increase the patient's role in determining the nature of therapy information disclosed, Roter (1977) primed and rehearsed question-asking with patients in the waiting room prior to their appointment with the doctor. Results indicated that while the number of questions increased, patients were less satisfied with the visit and experienced more negative affect (anger and anxiety) during the visit. Evidently, when placed in the role of initiating discussion, patients obtain more of the information they desire but at an emotional cost.

Several studies have used modeling interventions to increase question-asking. Anderson, DeVellis and DeVellis (1987) showed patients video tapes of model patients who either asked questions or revealed problems. Subjects who saw the question-asking video tended to verbalize more and sooner in the health care interaction. Greater patient verbalizations were correlated with increased satisfaction but there was no difference between modeling or control (no video) conditions in patient knowledge scores.

Tabak (1988) provided patients with a booklet containing sample questions that they could use as a basis for asking about their own care. Although there was a 32% increase in question asking in the experimental group receiving the booklet compared to a group that did not receive the booklet, the difference between groups was not statistically significant. Examination of the question asking distribution indicated that the mean number of questions asked by patients was quite small, with a small number of patients who received the booklet asking a large number of questions. Thus, this intervention may be viable with only a select number of patients.

Robinson and Whitfield (1985) used a less invasive technique to prime question-asking. They compared a "permission" group (merely telling patients that the doctor would be happy to answer their questions) and a "guidance" group (patients were asked to imagine carrying out the doctor's instructions and to raise questions about problems that might arise) to a "normal" group that was not given any special instructions. There was no difference between the normal and permission groups; however, the guidance group asked more questions and had more accurate knowledge of the therapy. Interesting, there was no difference between the groups in their own reports of understanding of the physician's instructions.

If patients understand how information is to be used, they may make better judgments about what they need to know. In the Glenberg, Sanocki, Epstein and Morris (1987) study, better "calibration" of knowledge was obtained when people were provided with a criterion test that provided a more precise basis for comprehension. Thus, if patients understand how they will have to use the information (e.g., what decisions need to be made, what behaviors need to be enacted) they may be able to make better judgments about the relationship between their informational base and the information they need to know.

There are at least two important insights gained from these question-asking studies. First, asking the doctor questions about treatment is not simply a cognitive exercise; there are potent emotional considerations as well. When patients start initiating questions about their treatment, they can become anxious and angry. The reason for this emotional reaction is unclear. It may be due to placing patients in an uncomfortable relationship with their physician, it may be due to fostering an increased perception of the risks undertaken by using the medication, or it may be due to forcing patients to realize the extent to which they have been uninformed about their treatment. Clearly, studies of patients' emotional reaction to risk information disclosures is warranted.

Secondly, the success of the "guidance" intervention in the Robinson and Whitfield (1985) study suggests that if information is to be communicated from doctor to patient, then how the information is incorporated in the patient's knowledge schema and behavioral plans is important. Patients seek to learn risk information for a reason. How the information is to be used determines what specific material should be communicated. In most therapeutic encounters, instructions about how to use drugs correctly is of most concern to the doctor. As patients' coping strategies are likely to change over time, the information presented about therapeutic risks needs to be reiterated in a modified fashion as discussions about the treatment continue over the course of the therapy.

While the studies cited above indicate that patients want to know a lot more about their medication (especially the risks of medication) it is unclear if it is reasonable to communicate that information during verbal encounters where the patient is trying to understand the cause and course of the illness. Risk information may be better solicited, understood, and applied when patients are actively planning behavioral coping strategies.

Increasing patient involvement

The extent to which risk information will be useful for a patient will depend on how relevant the information is to the patient's immediate needs and goals. Personal relevance, or "involvement," may be conceived either as a long standing orientation towards a product category or as a situationally stimulated motivational state precipitated by an immediate need (Zaichkowsky, 1985). The assertive "questioners" identified in the segmentation study may be representative of individuals who remain activated in their search for risk information across situations. Individuals who respond to the question-asking interventions posed in the studies cited above may be representative of people who are situationally involved with their therapy.

Research on consumer involvement with the products they utilize suggests that there are many different reasons why consumers become involved with particular products on a long term basis. Laurent and Kapferer (1985) found four independent factors that explained consumers' involvement with a wide range of products: the importance of the negative consequences of a mispurchase, the subjective probability that a product would be mispurchased, the emotional or pleasure value offered by the product, and the social or symbolic value of the product.

One may apply each of Laurent and Kapferer's factors to medical therapies to derive reasons why patients may want to learn about their treatments. The probability and negative consequences of a mispurchase are great. These products have a strong propensity for causing pleasure or pain. Medicines have significant emotional and symbolic value as they represent the hope of the patient and the power of the physician (Shapiro and Morris, 1978). The doctor-patient relationship is a potent moderator of involvement with treatment that often controls the extent of risk communication. This relationship is likely to moderate not only the patient's beliefs about the probability and severity of a "mispurchase," but pleasure and symbolic values of the therapy.

Situational involvement is usually conceived as a temporary motivational state triggered by the need to make a purchase decision (Zaichkowsky, 1985). Petty, Cacioppo and Schumann (1983) demonstrated that varying situational involvement (telling some subjects that they were going to make a product selection whereas other subjects were told the decision was not imminent) led to different sensitivities to promotional messages. Involved subjects (who anticipated making a decision) were more likely to respond to the quality of the selling message whereas uninvolved subjects (who did not anticipate making a decision) were more likely to respond to extraneous elements of the selling environment (the attractiveness of the product spokesperson).

As the physician usually selects products, decision making is often not a compelling factor for the patient in therapy. However, mastery and control motivation may temporarily stimulate involvement with the medication. Thus, if a patient is self-motivated by mastery and control issues, or if these motives are externally stimulated, risk information seeking may be increased. Greenfield, Kaplan and Ware (1985) stimulated patient involvement with their own care by having a clinic assistant review the patient's medical records and a treatment algorithm with the patient in a 20 minute session prior to the physician visit. The experimental patients were also encouraged to ask questions during the visit. Patients who received this counseling session were twice as likely as control patients to ask questions of their physician during the visit. These patients also indicated greater satisfaction with care, greater preference for a more activated role in medical decision making, and a greater adjustment to the disease.

It is clear that patients can be externally primed to increase their involvement with their own care. However, the manipulation applied by Greenfield, Kaplan and Ware extended beyond a mere motivational impetus, it also improved patient knowledge about the condition and treatment and reduced perceptions of environmental barriers by directly suggesting that the patient ask questions. From the question-asking studies cited above, it is clear that merely suggesting that patients ask questions is not sufficient for increased question-asking. Increased knowledge (knowing enough so a reasonable question may be formed) and the perceived need for information to fulfill mastery and control motives (the personal relevance of the information to help the patient learn how to respond to feared or anticipated problems) may also be necessary to improve risk information seeking propensities.

Making patients more situationally involved with their treatment may require a multitude of interventions to overcome the perceived costs of obtaining risk information. There appear to be fewer barriers for individuals who are involved on a long standing basis with their own care or with the medication they are taking. For these people, the physician is not the only source of information about the medication. They may be willing and able to consult additional knowledgeable sources (such as drug reference books). Furthermore, they may be more responsive to information they encounter on a continuing basis (e.g., magazine and newspaper articles) because of their long standing interest in the information. Beatty and Scott (1987) have shown that consumers with a long standing interest in a product category are more likely to consult neutral sources of information (consumer magazines) prior to making a purchase whereas consumers who were situationally involved were more likely to ask their friends about the product.

It is conceivable that stimulating situational and long term involvement are both viable strategies for improving risk information seeking. Interventions at the doctor-visit may initially have situational influences on risk information seeking but may also have ego-involving influences that remain over the long haul. The changes in patient attitude towards a greater role in medical decision making found in the Greenfield, Kaplan and Ware (1985) study were found one and one-half to two months after the involvement intervention. Thus, it is possible that once activated to seek information, and perceiving rewards for such activation, the patient learns the benefits of an active orientation toward risk information seeking. Secondly, public education that demonstrates the need to obtain more information about the risks of the therapies may have a stimulating role. Although public education cannot be as influential as direct experience in changing consumer's attitudes, the breadth of a public education program and its ability to reach people who are not in treatment is clearly advantageous. Obviously, both interventions will be successful only to the extent that they are fully supported, well planned, and thoroughly executed.

Implications

Examining the nature and extent of therapeutic risk information seeking, we see a great deal of patient passivity. In spite of much publicity about patient activation, actively seeking risk information seems to be viable for only a small segment of the population. On the other hand, patients seem to be greatly interested in obtaining risk information, willing to receive the information from a number of sources, and the beneficiary of a number of societal forces encouraging greater risk communication between health professional and patient. Although costly, interventions applied on an experimental basis could stimulate greater risk information seeking in everyday practice.

For the majority of patients, the physician controls the nature and extent of risk communication. The largest information seeking segment is composed of patients that are passively reliant on the physician for therapeutic advice. Therefore, to understand risk communications, a more complete understanding of the physician's orientation and behavior towards disclosing risk information is essential. We deal with this in the next chapter.

3
Physician's Risk Disclosure

As described in chapter two, for the majority of patients who receive therapeutic risk information, the physician is the primary source and additional sources are supplementary. Therefore, an examination of the nature and extent of physician delivered communications is essential to understand how patients learn about their therapies. Studies that have sought to measure the flow of information from doctor to patient have used a variety of methods. Unfortunately, measurement of this complex and dynamic interaction provides only limited insights that are correlated with the particular data gathering technique (Gerbert and Hargreaves, 1986).

In this chapter we will first explore what is known about the nature and extent of therapeutic risk disclosure based on observational studies and interviews with patients following the doctor-patient interaction. Unfortunately, methodological weaknesses and the lack of focus on the content of the interaction do not permit solid conclusions about the level of risk disclosure provided by the doctor. Furthermore, these descriptive studies do not provide a standard for judging whether observed levels of disclosure are sufficient. The chapter will also explore factors that moderate the disclosure of risks. It is hypothesized that physicians develop a "script" that determines what information is disclosed to patients about commonly prescribed therapies. Factors relating to the physician and the prescribing environment will be described that influence the execution of the script.

Normative Studies of Doctor-Patient Communication

Observational analyses

Several studies have directly observed or recorded physician-patient encounters and catalogued the information exchange. Initial studies used standardized systems, such as the Bales System (Smith, Polis and Hadac, 1981; Davis, 1968; Korsch and Negrette, 1972). A number of generalizations and potential barriers to communication were identified in these studies. It was found, for example, that interview length correlated positively with patient satisfaction and that physicians solicit information from patients to a greater extent than they provide directions. However, the rigidity of the cataloging systems and the large degree to which the systems focused on describing the process rather than the content of the interaction did not permit a full analysis of the extent to which risk information was provided to patients.

More recent observational studies have utilized cataloging systems that more specifically focus on a particular aspect of the physician-patient encounter. A number of studies have focused on the emotional or instructional aspects of the clinic visit. For example, Carter, Inui, Kukull and Haigh (1982) found that behaviors indicative of patient tension were negatively associated with satisfaction whereas tension release behaviors had a positive association. The timing of events within the encounter was also related to patient satisfaction. If patients requested medication therapy early in the interview and physicians were able to address the request and provide instructions later in the interview satisfaction was higher compared to situations where patients requested medication later in the interview and physicians could not fully explain reasons for granting or not granting the request.

Recently, Hall, Roter and Katz (1988) completed a meta-analysis of 41 studies that directly measured (through observation or recording) physician communication in the medical encounter. Several broad generalizations are possible from this analysis. Over all, the more information provided by the physician, the more satisfied and compliant the patient. The more information provided by the doctor, the more total information recalled by the patient but the less recalled as a proportion of the advice given. Patients of higher social class received more information than lower class patients, as did female and older patients. Physician questioning of the patient was negatively related to patient recall but physician efforts at "partnership building" (equalizing role relationships with the patient) were positively related to recall.

Although general reviews provide broad insights, it is obvious that the degree to which observational studies provide measures of the communication of therapeutic risks determines the usefulness of the study in understanding physician provision of risk information. The most direct measure of the content of therapeutic advice in the doctor-patient encounter is provided by Svarstad's (1976) study. Direct observations were made of 153 adult patient-visits to physicians in a neighborhood health clinic in the Bronx, New York. Svarstad concentrated on the nature of physician instructions regarding prescribed medication. Of the 347 drugs prescribed, explicit verbal advice on the length of use was provided in only 10% of the cases and frequency of use was discussed in only 17% of the cases. In 29% of the cases no information was provided about the drug's purpose and in another 17% the drug was never mentioned. Although Svarstad's study is the most focused in this area, the characteristics of the patient population and datedness of the study make the low degree of risk communication somewhat suspect.

Patient interviews

A second method of measuring physicians' communication relies on patient recall of the content of the interaction. Due to the frequency with which medication instructions are delivered in the doctor-patient encounter and the ease with which this particular set of instructions may be measured in a personal or telephone interview, several studies have measured patient recall of drug information.

Studies in the mid-1970's found a startling lack of therapeutic advice provided to patients by the doctor or the medical staff. In a telephone survey, Hoff (1975) found that 48% of 415 respondents said they did not talk to their doctor when their most recent prescription was written. Nickerson (1972) found that 65% of patients discharged from a Massachusetts hospital said that they were given no specific discharge instructions about their therapy.

More recent studies, such as the Morris, Grossman, Barkdoll, Gordon and Soviero (1984) study, find somewhat greater levels of therapeutic advice provided by doctors. Most patients (70%) said they received some information at the doctor's office; a little over half (about 60%) said they received directions for use information, about half that number (32%) said they received precautionary information, and information about side effects was delivered at a somewhat lesser rate (26%). In a recent study of clinic counseling Gardner, Rulien, McGhan and Mead (1988) asked 70 HMO patients who were waiting to have their prescription filled what information the doctor had provided during the visit. Approximately two-thirds indicated they had received information about the purpose of the medicine (67%), when and how much to take (64%), precautions (60%), and duration of use (59%); whereas less than half indicated that they received information about side effects (40%), drug interactions (17%), food interactions (24%), or what to do about side effects (17%).

The increased rates of therapeutic instructions and risk information found in HMO patients may be indicative of a patient segment that is both knowledgeable about and interested in health issues. Doctors may be more willing to share therapeutic risk information with these patients, especially precautionary advice.

Although care must be exercised in generalizing the results of HMO patients to the larger population, we may conceive of the HMO environment as a microcosm capable of predicting future trends in health care. The conflicting pressures on the professional staff caused by a changing demographic and psychographic base of patients that more actively seek risk information and the pressures to hold down medical costs are highly evident in the HMO. The Gardner, Rulien, McGhan and Mead (1988) study suggests that the increasing knowledge and interest of patients may do more to stimulate therapeutic counseling than efforts on cost containment to keep the therapeutic encounter as brief as possible.

The direct observation and patient interview studies provide differing insights into the content of risk disclosure in the doctor-patient interaction. However, several methodological problems make interpretation of these studies tenuous.

Performing direct observation and audio or video recordings are highly contingent on the cooperation of physicians (Cartwright, Lucas and O'Brien, 1976). Non-random samples of physicians may reflect results from patients attending clinics or receiving treatment from academically-oriented physicians. Obtrusiveness of the measuring device is an obvious problem, although patients and physicians may adjust to the measuring device as the interaction proceeds (Starfield, Steinwachs, Morris, Bause, Siebert and Westin, 1981).

Studies that rely on patient recall are highly suspect because of the frailties of human memory. As with memory for any interaction, patients may forget whole classes of information delivered in the interaction and have great difficulty remembering details. A recent study by Stafford, Burggraf and Sharkey (1987) indicates that people can recall only 10% of the "thought ideas" from casual conversation when interviewed immediately and only 4% when interviewed one month later. Alternatively, patients may report receiving information that is logically consistent with what they believe should have been delivered but was not actually provided. Studies of eye witnesses' report of dramatic events suggests a great deal of "creativity" in human recall when asked to refabricate details of an event (Loftus and Palmer, 1974).

Information Exchange Standards

Although much of the data bearing on physician disclosure of risk information can be criticized on methodological grounds, the percentage of patients who are informed about risks, or claim to be informed, is consistently less than half of the patient population. It is difficult to attribute these disclosure levels to methodological difficulties alone. One must assume that low levels of risk disclosure represent the norm for the patient groups studied.

On the other hand, conclusions about low levels of disclosure are made in an absolute sense, without reference to any standard.

How much and what specific risk information should be communicated to patients? How much can we reasonably expect patients to remember, interpret correctly, and use to guide their health care behavior? One may appropriately ask about the "quality" of doctor-patient communications rather than its "quantity" by examining the extent to which the important risks of treatment are communicated to patients.

A recent study by Tuckett, Boulton and Olson (1985) suggests that the communication of important concepts about drug utilization may not be as poor as indicated by prior research. Recordings of 328 British doctor-patient consultations were reviewed by an independent judge and key messages in the consultation were identified. Patients were then interviewed in their homes and asked to give an account of the consultation. Only 3% of the patients could not recall the key points made by the physician. Patients in the study were also asked to provide their interpretation of the doctor's advice (could the patient correctly understand the meaning and significance of what the doctor had said) and their commitment to following the doctor's orders (did they agree with the doctor and were they willing to follow the treatment plan). In only 8% of the cases were the doctor's suggestions misinterpreted but in 21% of the cases the patient was judged to be uncommitted to following the treatment plan.

The Tuckett, Boulton and Olson (1985) study stands in stark contrast with similar studies which have interviewed patients after the physician consultation and found poor recall (usually less than half) of the instructions, especially treatment and risk information (Anderson, Dodman, Kopelman and Fleming, 1979; Brody, 1980; Joyce, Caple, Mason, Reynolds and Mathews, 1969; Ley, 1978). The major difference between the Tuckett, Boulton and Olson (1985) study and the other studies lies in the standard used to define adequate recall. Evidently, patients can recall and correctly interpret only a limited number of "key" points from a conversation. Using a relatively low standard (what is identified as important from the information that a physician discloses) leads to higher communication scores than an a priori standard (what experts may agree is important information) or a standard based upon what the patient wants to know or believes is important to know (Faden, Becker, Lewis,

Freeman and Faden, 1981; Columbia Broadcasting System, 1984). The Tuckett, Boulton and Olson study also begs the question of whether the physician's directions are sufficient to achieve reasonable education goals.

Risk Disclosure Factors

In addition to examining descriptions of the doctor-patient interaction, we can also learn about risk communication by examining factors that moderate the physician's disclosure of risks. For example, in addition to measuring the content of the interaction, Svarstad (1976) analyzed the conditions which favored or inhibited the disclosure of drug information. One important insight gained from this study was the manner in which time pressure on the physician (as operationalized by the presence of other patients in the waiting room) influenced the physician's disclosures. Svarstad found that time pressures reduced the flow of information only if the patient had taken the prescribed drug on a previous occasion. Furthermore, when a drug was discussed with a patient it tended to be discussed "fully" (disclosing all the information the physician believed important).

Evidence of consistency in physicians' therapeutic counseling is also provided in a study by Hall, Roter and Katz (1987). The authors recorded and coded the therapeutic encounters between physicians and two "patient simulators" presenting symptoms for two different chronic obstructive pulmonary diseases (bronchitis and emphysema). Correlations between patient encounters for each of the 41 physicians showed a high degree of similarity in the delivery of medical information ($r = .57$). Even though physicians differ in the "style" of communication, for similar diseases, physicians appear to have a generalized tendency to provide a set amount of information in a prescribed fashion.

Based upon Svarstad's (1976) and Hall, Roter and Katz's (1987) results, we may postulate that physicians have a "script" that they repeat for each of the drugs they commonly prescribe (Bower, Black and Turner, 1979; Bower and Clark-Meyers, 1980; Yekovich and Walker, 1986). Once a therapy is chosen, physicians have an expected series of statements that they deliver to the patient about the therapy. Over time the script is formed and polished based upon feedback from patients. With time the script becomes well practiced and available in memory whenever a patient is prescribed the particular therapy. Whether or not physicians articulate the script is dependent upon cues offered by the patient that the information is necessary (or will be effective if delivered) and situational demands. From Svarstad's study we may presume that physicians will execute the entire script if there are no time pressures but if such pressures exist they will forgo it only if the physician believes that the patient can utilize the therapy correctly without such information.

Physician's script

Review of therapeutic risk information disclosed in the doctor-patient interview, therefore, needs to focus on: (1) the information contained in the routine script that physicians utilize, (2) how different physicians learn and modify the script, (3) how the script is adapted for different types of patients and (4) important situational factors that determine whether or not the script is performed and influence how the script is modified to fit the occasion.

The most direct measure of the basic script routinely utilized comes from a study in which physicians were queried about the information they routinely provide to patients about prescribed medications. Boyle (1983) asked a national sample of physicians to describe what information they normally provide patients who had not taken the prescribed drug on a previous occasion. Information was solicited regarding four commonly prescribed medications.

For warfarin (an anticoagulating drug), 73% of the sample said they tell patients to look for signs of unusual bleeding and 51% mentioned drug (aspirin) interactions; for thiazide (an antihypertensive), 61% said they tell patients to take it with orange juice. No other cautions, warnings, or side effects were mentioned by more than half of the sample. Furthermore, there were no side effects or warnings mentioned by more than half of the sample for tetracycline antibiotics or for benzodiazepine tranquilizers.

Thus, by physicians' report, drug side effects are frequently not disclosed during the initial consultation. However, the Boyle study does suggest that physicians may phrase precautionary information in the form of instructions. In the patient surveys reported earlier, there were equally low levels of precautionary and side effect information reported. Boyle's study indicates higher levels of disclosure for precautions compared to side effects. Patients may interpret precautions as instructions for use. The study also suggests that physicians may be more willing to disclose risk information to patients if the information can be framed in a way to emphasize how to avoid or counteract negative therapeutic effects. There was little data in the Boyle (1983) study to indicate that physicians routinely disclose rare or unavoidable side effects to patients.

Clearly, we must expect differences among physicians as to what constitutes the proper script. Numerous factors are likely to influence "writing" and "execution" of the script, especially the degree to which risk information is included in the disclosure. We may discern some of the more influential of these moderating factors by virtue of whether they stem from the physician or from the prescribing environment in which the physician operates.

Moderating Factors - The Physician

Individual differences

Differences in the background, training and personality of physicians influences the degree to which risk information is included in the routine script. It is generally found that younger physicians spend more time communicating health information to patients (Roter, Hall and Katz, 1988). More experienced physicians tend to keep their visits shorter, perhaps to manage work flow more efficiently and to avoid providing information that creates problems in the encounter. On the other hand, younger physicians may experiment with different disclosure patterns, weighing their knowledge about a therapy with patient response, to develop a script that is both informative and efficient.

Physician specialty is a conspicuous correlate of risk disclosure, if for no other reason than differences in the risks associated with the therapies utilized. Surgeons and anesthesiologists may be used to dealing with therapies that require extensive risk disclosure whereas pediatricians and dermatologists may be inexperienced dealing with treatments that pose significant risks to their patients. It is also probable that physician specialty is correlated with differing perceptions of the genesis of the illness and required treatment (Ashworth, Williamson and Montano, 1984). Within the same disease category, specialists differ in the degree to which they perceive the patient as suffering from psychogenic or somatic complaints and choose different therapies based on these perceptions (Eisenberg, 1979). In one study of difficult to diagnose patients, internists tended to perform diagnostic tests, surgeons used placebos, and general practitioners prescribed psychotropic drugs (Carey and Dogan, 1971). However, it is unclear if specialty is a cause of this systematic difference in patient perception or a result of underlying values and personality characteristics.

Although operationalized in many ways, the personality variable that has been most often associated with physicians' interaction with patients is the degree of "humanism" portrayed by the physician (Linn, DiMatteo, Cope and Robbins, 1987). Generally, humanism can be understood in terms of whether the physician treats the disease or is sensitive to the patient as a whole person. This characteristic, interacting with the patient's diagnosis, is correlated with the physician's willingness to tolerate risks in their choice of therapy. For example, Staudenmayer and Lefkowitz (1981) found that patients who complained about their symptoms to a moderate degree were treated similarly by physicians who differed in their sensitivity to the whole patient. However, for patients who minimized or emphasized their complaints, "low sensitivity" physicians (i.e., less humanistic) used potent drugs and discharged patients sooner whereas "high sensitivity" physicians kept patients hospitalized for longer periods and used less potent drugs.

If a risky treatment is utilized, it is unclear how physician "humanism" relates to risk disclosure. If a physician discloses risks in an attempt to elevate the patient's status in the relationship, this may be due to a "humanistic" orientation. If a physician discloses risks to fulfill legal requirements or if it is merely perceived as part of the treatment necessary to make the patient well, then risk disclosure may be due to a more task orientated, less humanistic physician.

Svarstad and Lipton (1977) found that when physicians were willing to frankly discuss the diagnosis of mental retardation with parents of the patient, there was more acceptance of the diagnosis but lower levels of reassurance produced. Thus, a frank discussion of the risks of treatment may emanate from physicians who are willing to tolerate some degree of immediate patient dissatisfaction to accomplish treatment objectives. Physicians who tend to concentrate on the socioemotional aspects of the encounter, rather than the task of solving the patient's problem, may be unwilling to frankly convey the risks of treatment to the patient. Interestingly, patients generally are more satisfied with physician behavior that is task directed rather than socioemotionally directed (Roter, Hall and Katz, 1987). Therefore, willingness to discuss treatment risks with patients may require a high degree of goal orientation and ego strength as the physician may need to tolerate short term patient dissatisfaction for longer term evaluations based upon patient perceptions that the physician is interested in helping the patient face and solve problems of treatment.

Role and attitude
During the nineteenth century, physicians viewed themselves as the minister of hope and comforter to the sick. Bad news, which might be upsetting to the patient, was meticulously avoided. Family and friends were left the task of informing the patient of a negative prognosis or the untoward aspects of therapy (Reiser, 1980).

Today, medical ethics leads to the view that the physician's role and responsibilities is to more fully inform patients about therapeutic risks. Many believe in a "guidance-cooperation" reciprocal role relationship between doctor and patient or a more egalitarian "therapeutic alliance" (Barofsky, 1978; Szasz and Hollander, 1956; Thomasma, 1983; Brody, 1980; Quill, 1983). In these relationships, the patient shares with the physician the responsibility of following advice and there is a greater sharing of information about the disease and decision making responsibility about its treatment.

It is evident that physicians themselves have come to view their role as requiring less paternalism and decision making authority. One often cited illustration of how far physicians' attitudes have changed in recent years is the case of informing patients about the diagnosis of cancer (Klenow and Youngs, 1987). In 1977, 97% of physicians surveyed believed that patients with cancer should be informed of their diagnosis. In an identical survey 16 years earlier, 90% of physicians believed that the patient should not be told (Novak, Plumer, Smith, Ochitill, Morrow and Benettt, 1979).

Examining reasons for this almost complete reversal in physicians' attitudes about informing patients about cancer, Amir (1987) found that there was a complex interaction of motivation with the type of information disclosed. The physician's orientation towards informing patients was the major determinant of providing diagnostic information whereas perceptions of the seriousness of the condition was the major determinant of providing prognosis information. Thus, changes in perception of the physician's role, along with the notable improvement in cancer survival rates, has increased communication about the disease to the cancer patients. If physicians can provide a message of hope and give guidance for treatment, the physician is more willing to provide frightening prognostic information. The patients' rights movements, fear of liability, and the need for informed consent have doubtlessly contributed to a change in physician attitudes about the disclosure of risk information.

Even if physician attitudes have changed in recent years, it is evident that they still lag behind patients in the desire to share decision making responsibility. In a survey conducted by the American Board of Family Practice Physicians (AAFP, 1987), members of the general public and a sample of physicians were asked their perspectives of the doctor-patient relationship. A slight majority of the public (54%) perceived a good doctor as one who explains alternative treatments to a patient and lets the patient decide, whereas, a slight majority of the physicians (51%) believed that a good doctor is one that chooses a treatment and tells the patient what to do. Interestingly, a significant minority of both the public and physicians believed the opposite, so the diffusion of this attitude in both samples is incomplete. These differing attitudes also account for difficulties that physicians express attempting to understand patient perspectives. Physicians who believed in greater patient participation cite the need for patients to understand, participate, and comply with their treatments as justification. Physicians who believe in physician decision making cite the physicians' qualifications or lack of patient qualifications as justification.

Eisenberg, Kitz and Webber (1983) have shown that physicians' attitudes about shared decision making can result from their training. In their study, first year medical residents were given a questionnaire assessing views about decision making authority. Medical and surgical residents displayed similar attitudes when measured during this time period. During the third year of training the questionnaire was readministered. At that time, medical residents displayed the same attitude toward shared decision making but surgical residents had become more authoritarian. The authors concluded that the surgeons' change in attitude reflected a task oriented nature of their training.

Even if physicians perceive their role as "therapeutic guide," it is unclear if this translates to greater risk disclosure. Within this self-perceived role, it is the physician's responsibility to inform patients about how to use therapies correctly to avoid problems. Disclosure of unavoidable risks would not be perceived as a responsibility. Unless the patient is viewed as having a greater role in deciding about or consenting to therapy, serious and unavoidable risks are unlikely to be disclosed.

Although patients frequently indicate the desire for a greater role in sharing the decision making responsibility, it is unlikely that a shared decision making role would portray the common relationship between doctor and patient. Patients are unlikely to be willing to tolerate the deliberate and time consuming decision making processes that would be necessary to make decisions about mundane treatments. Vertinsky, Thompson and Uyeno (1974) found that when faced with the problem of a sore throat, most people preferred a "guidance-cooperation" role relationship model for doctor-patient interaction.

For more serious diseases and treatments, patients may, indeed, prefer a more active role in reviewing and selecting the therapy.

However, there is a serious inconsistency in patient perceptions compared to physician perceptions. Even within the guidance-cooperation role relationship, patients express a desire for information without expressing the desire to participate in the therapeutic decision making process. As discussed earlier, physicians tend to underestimate patients' desire for risk information outside of the decision making context (Strull, Lo and Charles, 1984).

Moderating Factors - Prescribing Environment

Many elements in the therapeutic environment modify the extent to which risk information is provided to patients. Although some of these factors are concrete and objective, most of the determinants of risk disclosure are based upon the physician's perception of reality, rather than the objective state of affairs.

In certain therapeutic situations, such as for surgery or when a hospital develops educational materials for routine distribution, the disclosure of risk information is institutionalized. Thus, informed consent procedures may require the health professional to disclose significant risks to patients undergoing certain therapies. We will review risk disclosure in informed consent environments later. For now, we will concentrate on situations where the health professional can control the nature and amount of risk information disclosed to the patient.

Disease and treatment

A primary determinant of the physician's disclosure of a therapy's risks is the physician's knowledge about the treatment. In addition, the physician goal in prescribing the therapy guides risk disclosure.

The precautions, side effects, and warnings incumbent in medical treatments are extensive. A casual reading of the **Physicians' Desk Reference** indicates there is an enormous amount of risk information available for the physician to know about each of the drugs approved for marketing. Many of these side effects are extremely rare while others are quite common. Even placebo treatments have side effects. Clearly, there is too much information available for the physician to know about each treatment's risks. The physician must learn the essential facts and discriminate the important signals from the concomitant noise.

The risk information that the physician learns and remembers is based upon how the physician intends to use the information. As most physicians learn a treatment's risks and benefits for the purpose of making therapeutic decisions, they will store a limited amount of information that will help them achieve this processing goal. To make these types of judgments, only the most salient and discriminating risk information is necessary (Tversky, Sattath and Slovic, 1988). Thus, given the purpose of having to make a decision about treatment, there is little incentive for physicians to commit large amounts of risk information to memory.

The way in which physicians learn about new therapies influences the amount of "new" information stored in memory. If the new treatment is unique or novel, the physician needs to perform an intensive review of the data. In this circumstance, the physician evaluates the information in a piecemeal, in depth fashion. If the therapy is similar to other "me too" treatments the physician processes the new information categorically. Only information on the new treatment that is different from existing "prototypes" or "exemplars" existing in memory are discerned. In this fashion physicians develop more individualized schema about innovative treatments and learn more extensive risk profiles for these treatments. Knowledge about risks for "me too" drugs is based upon existing schema for similar treatments. Risk information is generalized based upon the prototypes and exemplars.

Once a therapy becomes adopted by the physician, knowledge tends to accumulate with experience and feedback from the initial group of patients supplied with the therapy (Hoch and Deighton, 1989). One may expect common side effects, which are likely to be experienced by patients, to become part of the physician's active knowledge base and eventually to modify the physician's script for risk disclosure. However, rare side effects are unlikely to be reported by patients. Even if a therapy is prescribed frequently it is doubtful that many physicians would have direct experience with more than one or two, if any, patients who experience rare (one in 10,000 cases) adverse effects. Even if a patient experienced the adverse event, there is a strong likelihood that the adverse effect would not be attributed to the therapy or that the patient would visit a different doctor to treat the condition. If physicians base their knowledge about a therapy on their own experience, rather than scientific assessment and the published literature, it is likely that their knowledge is incomplete, especially as it relates to serious but rare adverse effects.

Regardless of how well the physician knows the treatment, the decision of what information to disclose to the patient will be modified by the physician's goal in the treatment situation. Diagnosing and treating the patient's condition is likely to be the physician's overriding concern. For humanistic oriented physicians, treating the whole patient and improving the patient's quality of life may be a major concern. Sensitivity to the patient's needs and the vividly recalled experiences of former patients are likely to frame the physician's goals when deciding what risks to disclose.

Patients with differing diseases are likely to have differing concerns and problems. Patients who are dealing with a great deal of pain are unlikely to worry about long term risks when their immediate needs are so apparent. Patients with fatal diseases are similarly unlikely to be worried about treatment risks. Physicians would appear silly to bring up inconsequential risks when dealing with patients who have these conditions. Patients with asymptomatic conditions such as hypertension, on the other hand, are often unconvinced that they have any real problem. A frank discussion of treatment risks might be seen as counterproductive since it could persuade people not to take a medicine that is medically necessary.

Efficiently and safely managing the patient's treatment is also a major concern. If the physician perceives that the patient will fail to follow the treatment regimen because of a bothersome side effect that would eventually go away with continued treatment, the physician may be more inclined to forewarn the patient. Similarly, potentially dangerous side effects such as dizziness when driving are more likely to be communicated to new patients. As previously discussed, precautionary advice that can be used by patients to protect themselves from harm is much more likely to be communicated to patients than serious, rare, and unavoidable risks.

Therefore, for each treatment, the physician is likely to learn, and choose to communicate, only those elements of the treatment's risks that are necessary to serve the perceived needs of the patient and achieve therapeutic and practice management goals. In a study of physician disclosure of surgery risks to parents planning to circumcise their infant sons, Christensen-Szalanski, Boyce, Harrell and Gardner (1987) measured which of the myriad of surgical complications were conveyed to parents. Parents were routinely informed of only a small minority of the risks. Selecting which risks to convey, surgeons apparently used some subjective assessment of the frequency and severity of the possible outcomes to make their selection. Neither the probability nor seriousness of the risks by themselves were compelling factors in determining disclosure. Unfortunately, physicians consistently regarded the seriousness of the complications as less severe than the parents.

Patient perception

What physicians tell patients will in large part be based upon physicians' perceptions of what patients want to know, how well they will be able to convey the information, and how patients will react to the information. Thus, the physician's perception of the patient is a critical determinant of what risk information will be disclosed. As doctor-patient relationships have become more fragmented in recent years, the physician's perceptions are likely to be based on a quick read of the patient rather than a long term association.

Models of social cognition suggest that the perception that physicians form of their patients will be based upon their information processing objective (c.f., Wyer and Srull, 1986). When first interviewed, doctors are likely to focus on those characteristics of the patient that help form a diagnosis. Biological (gender, age, body weight) and behavioral (lifestyle habits) characteristics are most critical in this regard. These elements along with directly observable characteristics (social class, verbal ability) are the major elements available to the physician to form an impression of the patient. Psychological and social factors (e.g., recent stressful events) are unlikely to be determined in the medical interview (Brody, 1980).

Once the physician has formed a diagnosis, it becomes an organizational construct that guides the input of additional information (Arkes and Harkness, 1980). Information that is consistent with the diagnosis and first impression will be remembered whereas inconsistent information is more apt to be forgotten. Inferences about patients and their problem stem from existing organizational constructs. The diagnosis also serves as a social label that guides interpretation of patient interactions. In a study of nursing students, patients without a definitive diagnosis were rated less favorably, and their pain was seen as less genuine, than patients with a clear diagnosis of a kidney stone (Gillmore and Hill, 1981).

From this imprecise data base, the physician may judge what risk information the patient wishes to know. When physicians search for direct evidence of patients' desire to know about the risks of treatment, they may mistakenly believe that patients do not really want to know about their therapy because they do not ask questions or seek clarifications. In making such a determination, the physician may take into account the perceived intelligence level of the patient. If the patient is perceived as intelligent but does not ask, the physician may be more assured that the patient does not wish to know the risks of treatment (Amir, 1987).

The physician's judgments about the patient's desire to know may also be influenced by ego defensive motives. In a British study, physicians of 279 patients who died of malignant disease were asked if they had told their patient the diagnosis and prognosis. Only 13% of the physicians said they did. However, 46% of the physicians stated that they believed that the patient probably knew anyway.

Even if the patient wishes to know, the physician may perceive many difficulties in explaining complicated risks. In a British study, doctors were found to volunteer more explanations about treatment to patients of a higher social class than working class patients (Pendelton and Bocher, 1980). This difference could not be explained by differences in diagnostic rates for the two sets of patients. One possible explanation is that physicians foresaw difficulties explaining the problem to certain patients and, therefore, decided not to discuss the issue. Another study of 480 physician-patient consultations confirms that there are notable differences between upper and lower socioeconomic groups in their knowledge of the diagnosis and treatment and in the pattern of advice provided by the doctor (Bain, 1977). Obviously, language difficulties will influence communication. Svarstad (1979) found that English speaking physicians attempted fewer communications to Spanish speaking Puerto Rican patients than English speaking patients of the same socioeconomic level.

Certain patients may have more difficulty understanding risk information than others. Unfortunately, physicians tend to underestimate patients' knowledge of their disease and its treatment (Kane and Dueschle, 1967; Pool, 1980) and their ability to comprehend medical vocabulary (Segall and Roberts, 1980). Therefore, physicians may overestimate difficulty explaining therapy to patients. Initial perceptions, reinforced by the patient's lack of questions, may lead physicians to believe that patients are neither able nor willing to understand the complexities of their condition and its treatment. Attempts to simplify by analogy and example may confuse patients even further or lead to "mental models" of the treatment that inhibit proper self care (Meyer, Leventhal and Gutmann, 1985). Thus, physicians may omit explanations in light of these anticipated difficulties.

Physicians' perception of their patients' intelligence and cognitive functioning is based on surrogate indicators such as social class and verbal skills. Although these indicators are likely to be correlated with medical sophistication and desire to know, they are not likely to be as sensitive an indicator as a direct test. A patient's initial reaction to general or nonthreatening treatment information may be the best predictor of willingness and ability to process risk information than more removed perceptions of sociological characteristics. Patient perception may be misleading because the patients' acceptance of risk information can be situationally determined by virtue of which aspect of the coping process (i.e., disease causality, mastery, or ego defense) the patient is currently focusing upon.

It should be noted that physicians do not necessarily wish to avoid patients who have difficulty understanding therapeutic advice. In a study of patient analogues, Gerbert (1984) found that physicians stated they would discuss therapy more frequently with patients who were perceived as incompetent. However, the additional time spent with the difficult to educate patient would be devoted to explaining directions for use rather than providing risk information.

Physicians may withhold information because they fear that its impact will have negative implications. The patient's reaction to bad news may produce serious emotional ramifications, exacerbating old problems and creating new ones for the patient and the family. In the Christensen-Szalanski, Boyce, Harrell and Gardner (1987) study, one group of physicians was asked to verbally inform mothers about a full range of complications of circumcision. Several of the mothers were visibly uncomfortable after the 5 to 10 minute presentation of risk information and several of the physicians refused to participate in the study after a few tries at full risk disclosure. Reactions to rare but serious risk possibilities (e.g., uncertainty about the occurrence of cancer) can make long-term management of the patient difficult. By assuming that patients know the "bad news" without explicitly delivering it, the physician may rationalize an extremely difficult situation.

As shown in the Boyle (1983) study, common side effects, such as headaches, nausea, and stomach upset, may be left unexplained because the physician is uncertain about the possibility of the patient resisting therapy or developing suggestion induced side effects. The physician may believe that it is unwarranted to raise the possibility of problems when they might not occur or, alternatively, cause a problem to occur by virtue of a placebo effect.

A second type of uncertainty results from physicians' lack of definitive knowledge about the disease or its therapy. Under these circumstances, physicians may withhold information or provide only innocuous news rather than admit to their uncertainty. Reluctance to admit uncertainty may result from fear that: (1) patients will misinterpret the physician's lack of knowledge as an indication of a dismal prognosis, (2) patients will lose confidence in the physician if the physician appears out of control, or (3) physicians may lose confidence in their own ability to treat their patients' problems. The old adage "when in doubt - say nothing" provides the safest route when the physician is faced with a lack of information.

Situational factors

Any communication occurs within a broader context that helps define goals and establishes constraints that facilitate or inhibit risk disclosure. We tend to characterize situations in terms of the physical aspects of the environment and the people in it, social roles, feelings and personal dispositions, events that occur, the general atmosphere, and behaviors displayed (Cantor, Mischel and Schwartz, 1982). In addition, time factors influence risk disclosure (Christensen-Szalanski and Northcraft, 1985).

The physical facility in which the examination, interview, diagnosis, and treatment takes place controls risk communication patterns to a great extent. Hospitals may require risk disclosure, and have institutionalized patterns for disclosing risk, as well as special resources (e.g., an advice nurse) that facilitate and enhance risk disclosure. In certain hospitals the head nurse may be designated as the individual to provide therapeutic instructions whereas in other institutions the pharmacist on the ward or another specialist may undertake that role.

The institutional setting also establishes and reinforces a sense of control and power for individuals. Therapeutic communications occur most frequently in environments controlled by health professionals. The health professional determines when the patient will be seen, for how long, and what physically happens to the patient. It is difficult to ask the physician questions when the physician physically exits the treatment room, leaving the nurse to explain the therapy to the patient (Morris, Grossman, Barkdoll and Gordon, 1986).

In an interesting study by Sankar (1986), medical students were queried about communication problems that they experienced treating patients in their homes rather than at the clinic. The students mentioned a great number of difficulties stemming from changes in both physical and sociological parameters. For example, as patients had lower beds at home than in hospitals, the physician had to decide whether to sit down (and if so, on the bed or next to it) or stand up a far distance from the patient. As there were no supporting staff, the physician needed to solicit information from the patient directly. Family members were much more assertive, forcing physicians to pay attention to the patient, conforming to how they believed the physician should act.

We postulate that physical aspects of the environment may "cue" script variations. As physicians become more experienced, their script becomes enriched, adding contingencies (i.e., "subscripts") that adapt to environmental variations. Without this experience, the physician's script is less flexible. Physicians utilize the same script, regardless of environmental cues or patient perceptions. Svarstad (1976) found little modification in what advice was provided depending on whether the waiting room was full or empty. Nievaard (1987) investigated the influence of the "ward climate" on patient communications and found little association between the atmosphere and communications to patients. With experience, physicians may become more reactive to patient and situational cues that signal the need for script variations. Research on salesperson effectiveness suggests that more effective salespersons have highly developed, elaborated scripts that contain many variations adaptive to situational variations. There are relatively few major script categories, but many contingencies in the basic script (Leong, Busch and John, 1989).

Implications

For the most part, we expect that physicians, like any of us, become very "good" at what they do. For therapies that they utilize frequently, the disclosure of risks becomes scripted. With experience, the script becomes richer as the physician learns to adapt to new patients and circumstances. If it is true that younger physicians spend more time communicating health information than older physicians (c.f., Roter, Hall and Katz, 1988), then we must conclude that risk communication scripts are shortened with time and experience.

Boyle's (1983) study suggests that there may be more risk communication provided to patients than disclosed in studies that rely on patient memory, with physicians disclosing risks in terms of behavioral precautions (actions to take while using therapy) rather than risks of using a medication. It is unclear how phrasing risks as directions for using a treatment influences the patient's perceptions of the therapy or subsequent cognition, attitudes, or behaviors. In the next chapter, we will examine how the patient processes information about therapy, including risk information, to begin to explore how physicians' communications influence the patient.

4
Patient Information Processing

The verbal or written disclosure of risk information is dependent upon the health professional. However, the patient cannot be totally passive. To be successfully communicated, not only does risk information need to be disclosed, but it needs to be attended, understood, integrated, remembered, and ultimately put to proper use when decisions are made and behaviors undertaken. Even if emphasized by a physician, the patient must be able to fully process risk information for it to be of value.

Unfortunately, our ability to process risk information is necessarily limited and selective. With the myriad of complex environmental events ongoing at any time, human beings must be able to meaningfully discern and quickly react to only the most important ones. Much potential information becomes ignored or superficially examined because we do not have the capability to fully process all the stimuli in the environment. Our cognitive resources are conserved and applied to process those stimuli that are needed to achieve internally motivated or environmentally driven goals.

Adapting McGuire's (1980) model, we may conceive of risk communication as a series of stages through which any message to which we are exposed must pass in order to be fully processed. These stages frame the outline for this chapter as we review how the patient: (1) attends to and selects information elements within the communication, (2) decodes and meaningfully comprehends the selected messages, (3) integrates the new information with existing information in memory to form new knowledge structures, and (4) retrieves information from memory for later decision making or when self-protective behaviors are necessary. At each stage we will discuss

Attention to Risk Information

Merely paying attention to the doctor's therapeutic advice may be hard for patients. During the initial visit, listening to advice about therapy is difficult when patients are occupied worrying about the meaning of the diagnosis given earlier in the interview. At any time, limited attentional capacity is split between internal (self-generated) and external (environmental) stimuli. Furthermore, worrying divides the patient's attention and uses up some of the patient's limited attentional capacity (Eyesenck, 1979: Leight and Ellis, 1972).

Attention is the focusing of mental effort (Johnson and Dark, 1986). What we remember from the doctor's instructions is based upon our attentional focus during the visit. Varying attention levels while listening to different elements in the doctor's script selectively defines the internal information basis for patients' later decisions and behaviors. Understanding what patients pay attention to is, therefore, essential to understanding what elements within a conversation will serve as effective stimuli for patients' memory, decisions, and behavior.

Priming effects

Generally, attentional focus is guided by "priming effects," where one stimulus guides the processing of another stimulus (Johnson and Dark, 1986). Priming effects may be either "internal" or "external." Internal primes are linguistic cues provided in the conversation. These internal primes may be conversational elements that the patient believes are important for immediate or long term goals or they may be cues provided by the physician or the environmental context that guide how attention is focused (Kintsch, 1988). External primes are expectations that the patient has about what elements in the conversation are important. These external primes may be supplied by the doctor, some other person, or the patient's own beliefs.

The general information processing orientation that the patient brings to the doctor-patient interaction controls how limited attentional capacity is assigned. To overcome limits in attentional capacity, patients may adopt either a "bottom-up" or a "top down" information processing strategy. The strategy adopted not only influences what specific elements within the conversation are designated for fuller attention, but it also influences the information processing system at later stages and controls how fully each of the processed elements of the conversation are integrated into existing memory structures.

During the initial meetings, the patient often does not have firm expectations of what will happen during the visit with the doctor. Under these circumstances, information processing is likely to be "data-driven" or "bottom-up" (Kintsch, 1988). Without pre-existing ideas or explicit directions about what is important, patients may retain a "broad but shallow" focus on the conversation. With this broad focus, the patient attempts to understand the words, ideas, and concepts provided by the therapist. When the patient perceives that a certain element in the conversation is important, then that element becomes the focus of attention. Thus, the conversation itself (internal primes) rather than preconceived expectations (external primes) drives attention patterns.

If attention remains broadly focused on the entire conversation, it is likely that the patient will retain only a cursory memory of most of the conversation. This is because the broad focus does not permit deeper processing of any of the elements. We may conceive of information processing as proceeding at different levels (Greenwald and Leavitt, 1984). At the most basic level, the patient must provide a sensory analysis, hearing and recognizing the most significant words provided at the visit. Deeper levels of analysis require the patient to decode the message by understanding the individual words, integrating the words into meaningful concepts, and blending the concepts into personally meaningful knowledge structures.

Processing information through each of these progressively intensive levels requires greater attentional resources. The more we focus on one element in the conversation, the more selective we become about what is being processed. As attention becomes more directed, the more meaningful elements of the conversation are more fully processed, however; the other elements of the conversation are processed at lower levels of attention.

Certain aspects of the conversation may also influence the application of attentional resources. If patients are busy trying to decode unfamiliar terminology or if the precise meaning of the physician's directions is ambiguous and the patient must decipher the message using internal memory resources, it is unlikely that attentional resources will be available for processing other elements of the conversation. The patient may choose to ignore the more difficult aspects of the conversation. If, however, the patient believes that the difficult to process elements are important and worthy of attention, it will be difficult for the patient to process the other directions at more than the most cursory levels.

Given that patients are unable to fully process the entire conversation, the factors that control which conversational elements are more thoroughly processed become important. One would assume that the patient merely processes those elements within the conversation that are most important. However, lack of familiarity with the informational content of the interview makes the selection of elements for fuller processing subject to several biases.

With physician controlled conversation, the patient may not be able to understand important concepts. Therefore, ideas that the physician believes are important may be ignored by the patient simply because the patient does not immediately understand their significance. Physicians may believe that they are providing a relatively small number of important directions, assuming that patients would be able to fully attend to all of the directions mentioned in the script. However, the physician is likely to underestimate the difficulty that the patient has processing even the simple directions. Straightforward directions must be elaborated by the patient and additional "context" added so that the information will be personally meaningful. For example, if told to take their medication after every meal, the patient must think through contingencies such as how to carry the medicine with them to comply with instructions when eating out.

Patients may believe it would be ill advised to focus limited cognitive resources by attempting to think through the ramifications of simple directions risking inattention to other, perhaps more important and certainly more challenging, parts of the conversation. The Robinson and Whitfield (1985) study, in which patients were guided to "imagine carrying out the doctor's instructions" suggests that active elaboration of certain message elements (i.e., the doctor's instructions) increases certain behavioral responses (i.e., question asking). We hypothesize, however, that this focusing of attention on one aspect of the conversation leads to decreases in memory for other aspects of the conversation.

Given limited information processing capacity the patient may be highly selective in choosing which elements to elaborate. However, the patient may not know which elements in the conversation are important. Without internal primes, the patient may use linguistic cues as external primes to guide attentional focus. Unfortunately, normal linguistic cues may not apply to physician provided directions. For example, Ley (1972) found that patients tend to remember information presented early in the consultation, such as diagnostic information, rather than information presented later in the conversation, such as therapeutic advice and any discussion of the therapy's risks. When the order of the physician's routine directions was reversed, putting therapeutic advice first, patients remembered the therapeutic advice.

Under these circumstances, patients may direct their attention to those aspects of the physician's directions that are most familiar to them. Simply being exposed to a stimulus on a prior occasion enhances the ease with which it is recognized. This perceptual enhancement may lead the patient to concentrate on old problems, failing to recognize the severity of new problems. If new information is presented in a way that permits it to be logically attached to the previously learned material, the new material is more likely to be integrated in memory. It is easier to enhance existing memory than build new memory structures. A physician who provides information that enhances old information provides a better basis for learning. Thus, if a physician shows how a new complication is related to an old problem (e.g., a new symptom of diabetes, a side effect of existing therapy) rather than treating the condition as an entirely new problem, the patient may find the information easier to process, requiring less attentional capacity.

Thus far, we have assumed that the patient enters the physician-visit as a "blank-slate," letting factors within the visit prime attention. The CBS (1983) survey suggests that patients would be externally primed to attend to risk information. From an evolutionary and self-preservation viewpoint, risk information would be important for survival purposes. However, even if primed to be sensitive to therapeutic risk information, the physician, by phrasing risk information in the form of directions, embedded in a series of directions, may present the risk information in a format that is difficult for the patient to identify as risk material. Thus, if a doctor tells a patient to take medication with food, the patient may not realize that the medicine may cause gastrointestinal upset and that the directions are merely a means of avoiding adverse effects. Furthermore, external primes may be driven by expectations rather than desires. While patients may be interested in risk information, they may not expect to receive it during the initial doctor visit.

One method of improving risk communication would be to provide explicit external primes for the patient. If the physician tells the patient what is important and what the physician wants the patient to attend to, one would expect improved risk communication for those elements with some loss of knowledge about the other elements. Clear learning objectives, clearly communicated, would help patients know what subject matter is most worthy of their attention.

Comprehension

At the most basic level, patients often do not understand key terminology and instructions provided by the physician (Boyle, 1970; Riley, 1966; Samora, Sanders and Larson, 1961). Even college educated patients may have difficulty understanding certain terms (Tring and Hayes-Allen, 1973). For example, three-fourths of a sample of college students believed the term "pulmonary" referred to the heart rather than the lungs (Morris, Thilman and Myers, 1980).

Of course, patients do not need to understand each word a physician says to understand the important points. Problems arise, however, when patients fail to encode physicians' directions or encode them improperly, resulting in the failure of patients to understand the important implications of what is being said. For example, Korsch and Negrete (1972) reported that when a mother was told that her son would have to be "admitted for a work-up," the mother did not realize that the child would have to be hospitalized.

There has been much emphasis given to improving patient understanding of medical information. For example, numerous studies have been undertaken to measure the reading levels of medical information. However, readability tests have poor reliability and little consensual validation (Morris, Thilman and Myers, 1980). Information can be incomprehensible even if written at a low reading level (Bransford and Johnson, 1972). It is highly unlikely that short sentences, single syllable words, and limited vocabulary (the elements of most readability formulas that signify low reading levels) constitute sufficient conditions for patient understanding.

This emphasis on the structural elements of linguistic information seems misplaced. Stiles (1989) has suggested that a much more dynamic view of doctor-patient communication is necessary to provide a better understanding of how the process of communication leads to desired outcomes. Therefore, a more theoretically relevant basis of patient comprehension is necessary to define patient understanding. The degree to which the patient derives meaning from presented material provides a more meaningful indicator of patient comprehension rather than focusing solely on the presented material.

Context-availability model

The context-availability model provides a more complete framework for understanding what constitutes patient comprehension of medical information (Watenmaker and Shoben, 1987). The basic tenet of the context-availability model is that the comprehension process depends on the extent to which incoming information is attached to contextual information. Context is provided either from the material presented or from the listener's existing knowledge base. Comprehension is successful to the degree to which the patient is able to understand and establish relationships among concepts in the message.

The context-availability model suggests that medical vocabulary that is unfamiliar to the patient will not be comprehended because the patient will not be able to form meaningful associations between the new information and information that already exists in memory. However, if the unfamiliar vocabulary is explained, so that sufficient context is supplied with the new terminology, then the jargon may not only be understood, but may have other beneficial effects in increasing patients' comprehension (e.g., providing an organizational construct for future information). Thus, if the physician explains what would be involved with a "work-up" the patient may not only have insight into the meaning of the term, but would be able to relate the medical procedures that follow to a single concept, improving the patient's ability to remember and integrate the new information.

An important finding from research on the context-availability model is that "concrete" terminology (e.g., a scalpel), presented in isolation, is more readily understood than "abstract" terminology (e.g., a sharp instrument). However, when presented along with other material (in the form of a paragraph), there is no difference in understanding of concrete and abstract messages (Schwaneflugel and Shoben, 1983). Presumably, concrete information carries its own context whereas with abstract terminology the listener must supply the context to understand the relationships between terms. Unless new abstract information is sufficiently explained the listener may not be able to supply sufficient context to understand the message. The listener may make mistaken inferences about the meaning of the message because the self-generated context is incorrect.

From the above analysis, it is evident that the physician's use of vague terminology makes comprehension quite difficult. To save the patient from worrying physicians may use abstract terms (e.g., "there may be some serious side effects") and avoid concrete terms (e.g., "the treatment may cause a stroke"). The patient's lack of familiarity with the treatment may make it impossible to attach sufficient context to understand the meaning of the message.

The physician may also use euphemisms when presenting information to the patient. The word "elopement" means "escaped" in certain mental hospitals, "expired" means "death," and a "fussy" infant is one having a temper tantrum. Thus, the physician may avoid frightening the patient at the cost of causing confusion. If the patient attempts to supply needed context a good deal of confusion may result because of the patient's lack of familiarity with the treatment.

One of the major differences between the physician, as an expert in diagnosis and treatment, and the patient, as a novice, are the inferences that physicians make about the therapy compared to those of the patient. Inferences allow conversation to proceed without getting bogged down in minute detail. However, if correct inferences cannot be made then considerable confusion occurs. For example, if a physician tells a patient to eat chicken and avoid foods that are high in fat, the patient may believe that fried chicken is permissible unless the patient understands that cooking oil is a form of fat and that the oil is absorbed in the frying process. If the patient does not make the inferences that the physician intends, the patient may make incorrect judgments. Further, if the patient makes an incorrect inference, instructions may also be misunderstood. For example, if a physician tells a patient that a therapy may help "relieve" the symptoms they are experiencing, the patient may think that the treatment "cures" their condition when in actuality it is merely a short term therapy that allows the patient to rest quietly, and that bed rest is necessary for the patient to get better.

A number of commentators have advised physicians to avoid medical jargon to improve the comprehension of medical advice. However, the context-availability model suggests that important terminology can be effectively utilized if it is explained sufficiently. On the other hand, common euphemisms and abstract terms may provide barriers to comprehension because of the patient's inability to supply necessary inferences. Creating a script that contains specific terminology and sufficient embellishments to effectively communicate important risk concepts is an important step in risk communication.

Integration in Memory

To understand how the patient makes sense out of the information provided by the health professional, it is necessary to examine how the patient stores the therapeutic information in memory and integrates the material with existing information. Research in information processing suggests that memory is highly organized by virtue of how the individual perceives associations between informational content.

Schema

The basic organizational unit of memory is the "schema," where information is conceived as a series of "nodes" linked to one another in an association network. We may utilize several different types of schema to help organize and make sense out of the world. At least three types of schema have application to the communication of therapeutic risks and benefits. One type of schema is the "categorical" schema which serves to organize information about the environment and ourselves. A second type of schema are the "ad hoc" schema that are organized on the spur of the moment to solve problems we may have in understanding information or confronting issues. A third type of schema are "scripts" which contains a series of action sequences that the patient expects to occur in various situations. (We already discussed the physician's use of scripts for therapeutic discussions but will further elaborate on the concept below.)

Categorical schema: Categorical schema provide patients with a general orientation and perceptual basis for knowledge. We perceive and understand objects and events by placing them into categories. New information becomes associated with existing information already stored in our schema as we learn more about our world. How we organize these schema serves as the basis of how we perceive the world and is essential to our ability to communicate using a common (cultural) basis.

We are likely to have a schema for each of the major diseases that we learn about. Cognitive elements are associated with the disease and generally define our knowledge base. For example "hypertension" may be associated with the heart, blood, tension (anxiety), a blood pressure cuff, and water pills. In addition, emotional reactions, such as fear, may be incorporated (either in a symbolic form or by virtue of programmed physiological reactions) as well as visual elements (e.g., visions of an individual yelling loudly at his office mates). It should be noted that certain basic associations may be incorrect, as in the case that tension (anxiety) is not necessarily associated with hypertension.

The more an individual knows about a treatment, the fuller and more complete the schema. Schema are organized by virtue of their level of complexity, with basic organizational elements divided into numerous subordinate levels, depending on how thoroughly the concept is delineated (Meyers-Levy and Tybout, 1989). Although it is possible to build entirely new schema in memory, as described earlier, it is much easier to build new information into existing schema by attaching the incoming information to information already contained in memory. We can supplement the schema by accretion, adding new concepts to existing schema. Thus, if the doctor tells a patient that too much sodium is a cause of hypertension, "sodium" may become part of the hypertension schema.

Our knowledge base may change not only by adding new information but also by reorganizing existing information. If a schema is rich and full of associations, it may be "tuned" by reorganizing the schema into different patterns. If a schema becomes packed with information, the schema may be totally "restructured" as additional subordinate schema are developed and new associations (i.e., subschema) are formed. For example, we may develop a subschema for what causes hypertension (with subordinate levels for dietary causes, physiological changes, emotional reactions that precipitate it, and heredity) and another subschema for how hypertension is treated (with subordinate levels for medication, measurement of hypertension, and emotional reactions to treatment (visual and physical manifestations of fear)).

How therapeutic risk information is integrated into the schema is basic to how risk information is perceived. For example, as conceptualized above, fear is associated with the treatment rather than the cause of hypertension. Thus, we would expect this individual to react emotionally to the treatment and not the diagnosis. Associated information in the schema controls the meaning of the concept. For example, the extent to which risk information is integrated with benefit information in the medication section of the schema provided the basis for the patient's evaluation of the treatment.

The basic organizational structure and content of the schema determine risk evaluation. For example, rather than organizing the hypertension schema into subschema based on cause and treatment, it could be organized by virtue of environmental and physiological aspects of the disease. The patient could develop one subschema with environmental concerns (e.g., anxiety, sodium restriction, taking medication) and another subschema with physiological associations (e.g., visions of kidneys that do not function properly, how medications causes changes, exercise influences). If organized in this fashion it is unlikely that an assessment of treatment risks could be made without reorganizing the schema completely because the information about treatment is spread throughout the schema.

In addition to assessing information within the schema to make risk and benefit judgments, we may also look more broadly across schema to make comparative judgments. Thus, we may judge the riskiness of a disease by comparing it to other diseases. Diseases themselves may be organized conceptually into broad categories on the basis of a particular organizing framework. For example, Bishop (1988) has shown that college students conceive of diseases on the basis of "contagion" as a primary organizing principle. Therefore, AIDS is viewed as being similar to polio and malaria and distinct from lung cancer, stroke, and heart attack, which are viewed as similar to each other (life threatening but not contagious).

Ad hoc schema: We tend to organize information in memory on the basis of how we believe we will use the information. If we believe that we will need to make a decision between two forms of therapy, we may form separate schema for each alternative and store information in memory that distinguishes the alternatives. On the other hand, if we believe that there is no decision involved, but that therapeutic information will be used to control usage of the product, we may form schema based on behaviors necessary to use therapy properly.

Once a schema is formed to serve one purpose, we may later need to use the information for another purpose. In these instances, we spontaneously reorganize the schema to serve the new purpose. These new schema are created on an "ad hoc" basis. Reorganized schema that exist in memory permit us to solve unanticipated problems. If necessary, and if time and other resources exist, we may gather new information to supplement existing knowledge.

Ad hoc schema provide a great flexibility. We can use all the cognitive resources available to address unanticipated problems. Unfortunately, if the problem was unanticipated to begin with, the patient may not have paid attention to the original information to a sufficient degree to have a thorough memory for details. What was important for using a therapy properly (e.g., the dosage regimen) may have been unimportant for making a decision among treatments, whereas information germane to evaluating treatments (e.g., the risks and benefits of treatment) may be unattended during initial discussions.

Also, as unanticipated problems spur the formation of ad hoc schema, it is uncertain if therapeutic risk information will be perceived as relevant to the newly formed schema. For example, if a hypertensive patient is having difficulty because of frequent urination, the patient may search memory for information associated with this problem. If the patient does not associate hypertension or its treatment with frequent urination, then it is unlikely that therapeutic risk information (i.e., side effects of the medication) would be utilized to evaluate the problem.

The flexibility of ad hoc schema permits the development of cognitive structures that help patients understand medical treatments. When new information is provided, health professionals may help the patient organize the newly formed schema by informing patients how the information is to be utilized. This would tell the patient what organizing principles should be used to form the schema. Furthermore, providing patients with the general outline of a discussion prior to delivering the talk can help. In this way the patient can form a schema that efficiently organizes new information.

These "advanced organizers" (i.e., major schema organizing principles) have been shown to improve memory for medical information (Clarke and Johnstone, 1986).

Scripts: As described in chapter 2, a script is a sequence of directions. A script may also be formed to organize information about a series of expected actions. When a patient goes to the doctor, the patient expects certain events to occur in a prescribed order: sitting in the waiting room, going to the treatment room, being examined, having treatment explained, etc. If any of the tasks are not performed or performed out of sequence, the patient knows that something is wrong. The patient is not necessarily disappointed as patients may be pleasantly surprised as well.

The script that the patient holds for the doctor's explanations provides the basis for judgments about the success or failure of risk communication. If the patient expects risk information to be delivered, and it is not forthcoming, the patient has the basis for asking for the information perceived as missing. If, however, risk information is not part of the patient's script, and it is not delivered, the patient has no basis for seeking the information. It is not viewed as part of the script for therapeutic communication.

Elaboration

Integrating information in memory requires more than filing data into the correct pigeon hole. Risk information is likely to have many ramifications for the patient. It is vital to therapeutic assessment and may have important behavioral implications. To better understand the meaning of risk information, patients are likely to think about important risk messages, elaborating on their meaning and personalizing their implications.

This elaborative processing modifies the incoming information. Self-generated information is added to the schema and information that was initially stored may be rearranged depending upon the type of elaboration. Elaboration may also lead to the storage of information in additional schema as the patient thinks through the implications of the message.

Some elaboration may be necessary to make a conversation understandable. Simple inferences may be required to fill in gaps in the doctor's message. Other elaborations may entail substantive embellishments of the message when the patient makes extensive interpretations of the doctor's message, looking for meaning that may, or may not, be intended.

The extent of elaboration about therapeutic risks is likely to be determined by the "centrality" of the risk information to the patient's goals and values. Petty and Cacioppo's (1984) Elaboration Likelihood Model posits that people will elaborate on a message when they are involved with the information. In their study, Petty, Cacioppo and Schumann (1983) manipulated involvement by telling some subjects that they would need to make a decision based on information contained in a viewed message. Subjects who believed that they would need to make a decision paid attention to the message contents, whereas subjects who were not so informed were influenced by "peripheral" elements of the message (i.e., the attractiveness of the models).

We may assume that patients pay attention to selected elements within a longer message depending upon their level of involvement with those message elements. If the selected information is important enough, then the patient will elaborate those elements. However, uninvolved message elements will not be elaborated.

If the patient must make a decision about treatment, then risk information will be important and elaborated. Several different forms of elaboration are possible. The most common form of elaboration are embellishments that allow the patient to more fully understand the meaning and implications of what is said. Logical inferences are a common aspect of all communications. Unfortunately, the patient's lack of familiarity with medical matters may prohibit embellishments that the physician presumes will occur. For example, if a physician tells a patient to finish all the prescribed medicine the physician may assume that the occurrence of side effects would negate the physician's directions. However, patients may not make the logical inference that side effects would countermand the directive and maintain the regimen per the physician's directions.

The patient may "bolster" the risk messages by adding self-generated congruent implications. Bolstering can have an important outcome as the patient thinks through the ramifications of treatment risks. For example, if the patient is told that a surgical treatment will reduce fine finger movements, the patient may need to search memory to explore the activities that require fine finger movements in order to understand personal relevance of the side effect. As the patient finds activities that will be impacted, this new information would be stored in memory (e.g., I won't be able to paint on canvas, play the piano, or type my reports very quickly). Bolstering may also take the form of adding new information that is inferred from the broad context of the communication and from general knowledge that already exists. For example, the patient may infer that if fine finger movements are reduced that gross hand movements are also influenced, so that catching a ball or rowing a boat may also be more difficult.

If the patient believes that the risk information is a threat that is important to rationalize, then the patient may "counter-argue." When counter-arguing, the patient seeks to add arguments that dispel or limit the risks of treatment. For example, if informed about a reduction of fine finger movements, patients may counter-argue that, being in excellent physical condition, the side effects of the treatment are unlikely or will have little effect on their lifestyle. They may also perform some cognitive dissonance reducing strategy by assuming that painting and playing the piano are unimportant, that the secretary can provide typing services, and assume that gross motor movements would be unaffected.

In addition to counter-arguing, the patient may "derogate the source" of the message if the patient does not believe (or does not want to believe) that the message is accurate. Thus, the patient may simply elaborate on aspects of the source (e.g., the doctor is just out of school and not too experienced with my type of case). With the doctor as the source of the message, it may be difficult for the patient to utilize source derogation because of the perceived expertise of the physician and the increased dissonance this strategy would cause.

Processing Risk Communications

Both the physician and the patient organize information in memory using schema. However, vast differences in the expertise levels between the two parties make communication difficult. This difference between doctor and patient extends not only to the richness and organizational structure of their respective schema, but also to the way in which incoming information is processed.

The physician's familiarity with both choosing therapies and treating patients permits the physician to perform these tasks with much less cognitive effort compared to the patient. The physician can process information about the therapy in a "categorical" rather than a "piecemeal" fashion (Sujan, 1985). As experience grows, the physician can build mental prototypes for different types of therapies. These prototypes contain abstract images of the most common features of therapies. The more experienced the physician, the more sophisticated, complete, and finely discriminated these prototypes. When new therapies are encountered, the physician does not perform a feature by feature analysis of the treatment; rather the physician "examines" the therapy for distinguishing features and categorizes the new treatment into the most representative category. Thus, a new arthritis drug may be perceived as "another NSAID" (nonsteroidal antiinflammatory drug). Certainly, additional features are stored in memory that more fully describe the therapy and distinguish it from other members of the class. However, once the general categorization is made, the physician makes inferences about the safety of the medicine, as the risk profile of all NSAIDs are fairly similar and certainly different from other classes of antiarthritic drugs (e.g., steroids, gold salts).

Categorization also aids in emotional evaluation of the product. Fiske (1982) has suggested that prior experience with the category cues an affective response to new members of the category. Thus, categorization provides not only a set of beliefs, but may also provide a general orientation to "approach" or "avoid" the product category. If the category is seen as risky then new products may also be avoided.

For the patient, categorical processing may be possible in some instances if the patient is familiar with similar treatments. However, even if processed categorically, the mental representation of the therapy is likely to be based on a few "exemplars" (i.e., examples) that are less representative and less accurate of common features of the category. If categorical processing does occur, it occurs at a fairly broad level. The patient is more likely to characterize treatments on practical levels (e.g., all arthritis treatments) that are less theoretically relevant than the abstract level used by the physician (e.g., all nonsteroidal antiinflammatory drugs). Thus, the patient's ability to make inferences about the medication is reduced because many features related to the riskiness of the medication do not generalize very well across such a broad category. Broad categorization also establishes conditions where important mistakes can be made in risk assessment. If women taking Accutane merely viewed it as another acne treatment, they would be unlikely to infer that it had many risks (the drug causes birth defects if taken by pregnant women). For physicians, who may have viewed it as a "retinoid chemical" used for acne treatment, inferences about the risks of using retinoid treatments are correctly inferred.

If the therapy is unfamiliar (to either the doctor or patient) then "piecemeal" processing is necessary. Although doctors may need to use piecemeal processing for some novel and unique therapies, patients would be faced with these conditions on a much more routine basis. Under piecemeal processing, each important feature of the stimulus object is reviewed and an evaluation formed. It is also possible that some mixed models which combine categorical and piecemeal processing would be used by the patient (Cohen and Basu, 1987).

Feature by feature review of a treatment puts a large demand on the information processing system. The individual must store much more information to fully analyze a new treatment. Risk information may need to be "edited" in some form to reduce it to a more manageable level. Thus, the consumer may need to form an abstract representation of the "riskiness" of the treatment in order to maintain a coherent view of the therapy. Knowledge about individual risks may be summed to form an overall risk evaluation.

Information Retrieval

Therapeutic communications would be of little value unless the patient is able to retrieve pertinent information when necessary to make therapeutic decisions or engage in important behaviors. Clearly, all information presented will not be recalled. Attentional processes have already served to select only a portion of the presented information for storage in memory. Furthermore, not all the information that has been encoded in memory will be retrieved. Only information that is sufficiently "available" will be recalled.

It is generally believed that we become conscious of information in memory that has a sufficient level of "activation." We conceive of activation as a stimulation threshold. Unless a "node of information" located within a schema has a minimal level of activation, we will not be conscious of the material. Information becomes activated by external stimulation (recognition of words and pictures) and by internal search (activation spreads to associated concepts linked in memory).

When information is retrieved from memory, images and ideas are brought into consciousness. However, a full response (whether it be a verbal response, a conscious decision, or a memory response that triggers a behavior) requires combining the information retrieved from long term memory with situationally controlled information. Thus, we conceive of information retrieval as a creative process of refabrication. Studies of eye witness reports suggest that information reported to be retrieved from memory can be quite malleable depending on how questions are asked and what suggestions are made prior to the retrieval (Loftus and Palmer, 1974). To understand what information is retrieved from memory, therefore, requires an analysis of the content of information stored in memory, its activation level, method of organization, as well as situational factors that influence the search and refabrication process.

Only information that survives all the memory processes described earlier are subject to retrieval. It should be noted, however, that we are not passive recipients of information and that elaboration influences our knowledge base to an immense degree.

The more we elaborate on the risk information presented or self-generated about a therapy, the greater the likelihood that the risk information will be successfully recalled. There are several reasons why elaboration should increase retrieval. First, the more we elaborate on information at the time of input, the more we are likely to create multiple storage sites and association pathways. At the time of retrieval, activation spreads through associated concepts. Thus, there is a mathematically greater probability that the risk information will be retrieved simply on a probabilistic basis. Secondly, as we elaborate on presented information, we are likely to change the encoded message in several ways that increases its probability of retrieval. We may change the information to be more personally relevant. The recoded information more closely approximates conditions for retrieval because we have anticipated how the information is used and circumstances for retrieval. Thus, if the doctor tells us to take some medication an hour before bedtime, we may elaborate on that input by thinking of what we generally do an hour before bedtime (e.g., television shows we view). By drawing an association between the activity (i.e., the particular television show) and medication taking, the appropriate stimulus (i.e., the television show coming on) cues the pill taking behavior. Thus, by making the information more specific and self-relevant we increase the probability of recall.

Retrieving evaluations

Not only does elaboration influence the storage of information in memory, but recalling information influences the memory trace. If we have retrieved information on a prior occasion, there is a strong likelihood that the information has been utilized and re-stored in a modified form. The first time we form an evaluation of a treatment we must "construct" it on the basis of information stored in memory and situational factors. However, once the evaluation is formed, if asked again, we recall the prior evaluation. Thus, evaluations of treatment may be either "constructed" or "stored."

Stored evaluations occur with familiar therapies. The evaluation is based on internal memory operations and situational factors have minimal influence. However, constructed evaluations are based on the interaction of memory and situational factors. If we have never formed an evaluation of a treatment, we search for relevant information available in memory. The most easily recalled information is available and most influential in the evaluation process. The most recent experiences with the medication and the most vivid memory traces are apt to be highest in activation and most likely retrieved.

One of the most influential factors in retrieval is the precise "stimulus" that cues the memory search. Thus, in an informed consent situation, if the treating physician asks us for an evaluation of the proposed treatment, not only will we seek to recall all the relevant risks and benefits of the treatment, but information associated with the treating doctor is likely to be recalled. Information initially stored under different conditions (e.g., what we may have read about the treatment on a prior occasion) is more difficult to retrieve. This reduced availability is due to several factors: the passage of time between storage and recall; the lack of distinctiveness of the written word compared to information presented on an interpersonal basis (i.e., there are both visual and verbal memory traces encoded as well as more emotionally stimulating factors); the environment in which the information presented is different from the recall environment (i.e., with information presented by the doctor, the environment (e.g., the doctor's office) is the same under storage and recall conditions thereby forming stronger associations between storage and recall). There are also several biases in recall based upon how the evaluation question is posed. The evaluation process and its ramifications will be discussed in the next chapter.

Implications

Our information processing system is highly limited. The breadth and complexity of the information potentially available for assimilation about the therapies we undertake is beyond the capabilities of most patients to comprehend. However, our information processing system is remarkably flexible. We can approach information from a number of perspectives that permit either a broad (but shallow) or a focused (but limited) review of the data presented to us. Which perspective we take depends on our goals. Generally, we start out broadly focused and narrow our attention as we learn more about the information domain.

Given this forest of unfamiliar and potentially threatening information, how can the health professional best guide the patient? First, it appears that the patient's goals must be understood by the health professional so that the information presented is in concert with what the patient needs. Giving the patient an overview of the information to be provided during a counseling session may help the patient zero in on the most important elements in the conversation. Normal linguistic cues, such as viewing the initially presented information as the most important, simply may not work (Ley and Morris, 1984). Finally, as goals change over time and as patients learn more about their therapy, the long term relationship and continued discussion of therapeutic risks is important. The health professional must learn that risk communication is not a "one shot" occurrence. The risks of treatment may need to be addressed as the patient continues to take a treatment, confirming that the important risk information is integrated in basic knowledge structures and that the patient has elaborated on initial risks in ways that leave realistic memory traces.

5
Patients' Medical Judgments

Weighing risks and benefits to form a decision about the desirability of a therapy is inherent in the physician's role as prescriber. However, as discussed previously, the patient's desire to know risk information may reflect a need for anticipatory coping as well as meaningful participation in the therapeutic selection process. It is no wonder that many health professionals view the conveyance of risk information as an undesirable legal intrusion that interferes with the practice of medicine (Taylor and Kelner, 1987). When the patient is faced with the possibility of severe consequences from a disease or a therapy, it is natural for health professionals to assume that reassurance is necessary rather than the accurate transmission of risk information.

However, reassurance cannot fulfill the objectives of risk communications. Even if reassurance is indicated, ethical constraints and other objectives necessitate clear communication of therapeutic risks. In this chapter we will organize and discuss these other objectives underlying risk communication as stemming from the need for patients to make a *choice* among therapies, signify their *consent* to undergo treatments suggested by the health professional, and as a persuasive device used to improve *compliance* with directions provided by the health professional.

The Patient as a Decision Maker

Regardless of the patient's desire to participate in selecting a therapy, there are situations where the patient, and not the health professional, has greater "expertise" about the "issues" underlying the choice and is most qualified to make a proper choice among options. In these cases, the selection among therapeutic options is based on nonmedical factors and must rely on patients' perspectives of the therapeutic alternatives (including nontreatment) and their willingness and ability to deal with the problems created by the medical condition and its various treatments. For example, in selecting forms of birth control, the risks of using different forms can be stated in terms of medical outcomes; however, benefits cannot be stated in terms of the consequences of a disease or prevention of medical problems. Rather, the benefits of oral contraceptives, condoms, IUDs, or sterilization are based upon very personal views about the value of certainty of the birth control apparatus or procedure, ease of use, interruption of the lovemaking sequence, and permanence of the effects. These are very personal issues that can only be evaluated by patients themselves.

We may conceive of "elective" medical procedures as those where there is no medical justification for the treatment. Rather, therapy is undertaken to change physical stature or functioning. Clearly, in these circumstances only the patient's value system can be used to justify undertaking the risks of treatment. Elective procedures necessitate the active involvement of the patient in agreeing to the therapy.

Patient choice is also at issue in cases where the medical risks of treatment are so low that they may be almost nonexistent. However, financial or social risks may be quite great. For example, for the patient wishing to use Minoxidil as a hair restorer, there are few medical risks. However, the costs of maintaining a treatment regimen for the several months needed even to evaluate if the drug will be effective are great. Only patients can determine if the cosmetic benefits are worth the financial costs of the treatment.

In certain diseases, the risks among the treatment alternatives cannot be evaluated along a single, concrete dimension. Rather, due to the diversity of treatments, it is necessary to convert the concrete outcomes of each treatment to "abstract" dimensions permitting a comparison among the possible treatments (Johnson, 1988). In these instances, the patient is better able to judge the desirability of each treatment because the abstract criteria are understandable to the lay person. Furthermore, these abstract dimensions may only be evaluated relative to the patient's personal value system. For example, some cancers can be treated by radiation, chemotherapy, or surgery. The risks of all three are great, however quite diverse. How does one compare the consequences of being burned, losing a limb, or suffering the severe side effects of chemotherapy? Similarly, the benefits can be assessed differently depending upon whether survival rates are calculated as immediate or on the basis of living for five years after treatment (McNeill, Weichelbaum and Pauker, 1978). In these instances, there is increased interest in evaluating therapy in terms of the impact of treatment on the patient's "quality of life" (Morris, 1989). In addition to measuring the medical consequences of treatment, the impact of the treatment on the patient's physical functioning, mental health, every day functioning, social and role activities, and general perceptions of well being may be assessed and used to evaluate options (Ware, 1987).

In instances where patient choice is necessary, the patient (or the patient's agent) must make a decision. How these decisions are made and the degree to which they are free of external bias has been a matter of ethical debate for many years (Abram, 1982). To examine these issues, we must first explore the processes that patients utilize to make therapeutic decisions under conditions of risk and, secondly, examine the biases that can influence these decisions.

Decision making processes

As medical decisions invariably involve issues of gains and losses, analyses of patient and professional decision making have focused on how the critical trade-offs among therapies' benefits and risks are evaluated by the decision maker. Formal decision making models have been proposed that provide logical, systematic bases for optimal decisions. By using these models, we may analyze the expected utility of various courses of action and then choose the therapy that conforms to our most valued goals (c.f., Pauker, 1976).

However, these systematic models fail to account for how people process risk information, the contextual factors that may influence decision making, and how information is actually utilized (as opposed to how it should be utilized) to make decisions (Eraker, 1982; Diamond, Rozanski and Steuer, 1986). Although grounded in expected utility models, prospect theory (Tversky and Kahneman, 1981) provides a more thorough overview of the psychological factors and processes underlying patient decisions.

Prospect theory posits that there are two distinct stages in the choice process: an editing stage and an evaluation stage. During the editing stage the problem is analyzed initially and the decision maker structures the choice into a series of "prospects" or options. During the evaluation stage, pertinent information retrieved from memory is weighted, values are assigned to each of the options, and the option with the highest expected outcome is selected (Puto, 1987).

Editing stage: When first faced with a choice, the patient must review the options (e.g., surgery, chemotherapy, or radiation), their positive and negative effects, and other attributes or conditions related to each option. The options are apt to be provided and described by the doctor. More assertive patients may suggest their own options based upon general knowledge and/or seek second opinions to increase the number of options. The attributes related to each alternative are likely to be quite extensive and complex.

Given the complexity of the treatments, there are numerous criteria that may be used to evaluate each option. The patient is unlikely to have complete information on all these criteria. Furthermore, as stated above, the treatments may not be comparable on the most concrete criteria (e.g., chemotherapy causes nausea, radiation burns the skin, and surgery causes acute pain). Patients may be forced to recode and interpret these noncomparable alternatives on a more abstract level (e.g., the amount of discomfort expected). Due to the lack of complete information, the patient may need to make inferences about the performance of each alternative on the most important evaluative criteria. Certain vivid or easily interpreted outcomes may "signal" the performance of the therapeutic alternative on the abstract criteria (even if the patient does not understand what a particular term means). For example, if the patient is told that a drug causes "hyperkalemia" the patient may interpret it as a serious adverse effect.

Even with recoding many criteria to an abstract level, there may be too many attributes for the patient to fully process. Furthermore, each of these criteria must be weighted in some fashion for the patient to form an evaluation. At this point, the patient's goal in forming the evaluation is important. If the patient must make a selection among the options, how the patient views the end point in the selection process essentially controls which of the criteria will be valued and considered more completely. For example, people may choose to undergo one treatment as opposed to another for many possible reasons (e.g., to avoid pain, to please the doctor, to live an active life, to live longer, to maintain control of their own lives). Given these disparate goals, the selection of attributes is guided by which outcomes are most "diagnostic" or relevant to solving the problem. If pain avoidance is the goal, we expect that discomfort caused by the therapy is a major factor. If living a long life is the goal, survival rates are at issue. If remaining active is the goal then the disability caused by the therapy is weighted more heavily.

Evaluation stage: To form an evaluation based upon the "data" edited and stored in memory, the patient uses any of a number of decision making rules or heuristics. The decision may be based on a formal evaluation of the attributes, some simplification strategy that avoids active consideration of the attributes (e.g., do what the doctor says), or a global analysis that relies on the emotional factors. Numerous such rules may be operative for any given choice. Which decision rule or combination of rules is chosen depends on the goal of the patient and the particular circumstances in which the decision is made.

For example, a hypothetical cancer patient faced with the choice among chemotherapy, radiation, or surgery may utilize only a single criterion to decide what course to follow (i.e., the disjunctive rule). In this case, the patient decides to undergo surgery because it has the quickest outcome. Pain experienced and long term survival rates are not considered in the analysis. Another patient may reject all the options because they all are quite painful and disfigure the body (i.e., the conjunctive rule). None of the options surpass minimal criteria established by the patient for acceptable therapy. This patient may look toward an unorthodox cancer treatment because it is the only one surpassing the patient's threshold on the pain and disfigurement criteria. A third patient may consider the most important attribute first (which treatment is effective), then look at secondary characteristics (the pain levels produced), and then a third characteristic (how long will it take to undergo the treatment) (i.e., the lexicographic rule). Only therapies that are equal on each successive criterion are considered at the next level. Thus, radiation and chemotherapy may be considered equally effective and only these two treatments are analyzed for their painfulness. As chemotherapy is considered more painful, the patient selects radiation. Surgery, which may be the least painful was not considered on this attribute, having failed on the effectiveness criterion. A fourth decision rule that could be utilized is a compensatory rule, in which the consumer surveys the entire list of relevant attributes and averages out gains and losses on the basis of a weighted average (more important evaluative criteria are weighted more heavily). Although the weighted average approach tends to be used in subjective utility measurements and in predictive models of attitude formation (Fishbein and Ajzen, 1975), Tverksy, Sattath and Slovic (1988) have suggested that decisions involving the choice of one option over another tend to be made on the basis of a lexicographic rule, where evaluative criteria are considered successively. Decisions involving judgments of overall positive or negative evaluation (e.g., satisfaction with a treatment) tend to be based on a broader range of criteria, weighted in a compensatory fashion.

Biases in Decision Making

During the editing and evaluation stages, a number of factors may influence the decision making process to bias the choice. These biases may result from the way the information is presented to the patient or from the way people deal with the uncertainty of translating probabilistic information to make a personal choice.

Framing effects
Under conditions where the patient's goals are uncertain or conflicting, it is possible to stimulate certain of these goals through external means. The way in which prospects are introduced or "framed" (or the way patients frame the prospects themselves) has an important influence on decision making.

In some cases, people may see selecting a treatment as choosing among the worse of two evils. The exact same situation, viewed at another time and/or by another person, may be viewed as choosing the treatment that provides the best chance for success. For example, McNeill, Pauker, Sox and Tversky (1982) asked patients about their preferences regarding radiation or surgery as treatment for lung cancer. Patients' preferences for surgery differed markedly depending upon whether the life expectancies following surgical treatment were introduced in terms of the percentage of persons "living" as a result of the treatment or the reciprocal percentage of patients "dying" as a result of the treatment. Although the percentages in both cases were mathematically identical, preferences for surgery were markedly increased when patients viewed themselves as surviving the treatment.

The general finding from the risk perception literature is that people tend to be risk adverse when evaluating gains (a sure but moderate gain is better than taking a risk to win it all) and risk taking when it comes to evaluating losses (if I have nothing to lose, why not risk it) (Slovic, Fischhoff and Lichtenstein, 1985).

Framing effects are one of many factors that influence how individuals structure problems and edit information in memory. We may organize these additional biases in terms of how they influence the interpretation of risk information, the recall of risk information from memory at the time of decision making, and the evaluation and weighing of alternatives (Eraker and Polister, 1982; Morris, 1987).

Interpretation bias

As discussed in chapter 4, we interpret information in terms of the available context supplied with the message or inferred from our own memory. Risk information can be provided in either a relative or absolute sense. For example, treatment A can be 10 times riskier than treatment B. Clearly, treatment A is much riskier than B. However, we could have phrased the same information in an absolute sense; treatment A causes one death in 100,000 administrations, treatment B one death in 1,000,000 administrations. In this latter case there is little chance of a fatality from either treatment. The reference point provides patients with an "anchor" used to evaluate the risks. If we change the anchor, "adjustments" are made to reevaluate the risks because the comparison point changes.

If patients are not provided a formal anchor, they are forced to look for information to help them evaluate the risk in question. Rather than providing patients with absolute numerical statements of probability, physicians usually provide risk information in the form of adjectives. The probability of side effect occurring may be described as "rare," "improbable," "unlikely," "doubtful," etc. Even among physicians there is a wide variance in the interpretation of these terms (Bryant and Norman, 1980; Kenney, 1891; Toogood, 1980). Patients may not be able to supply sufficient "context" to interpret these linguistic statements with confidence. They may be forced to look for "signals" from the physician (e.g, gestures, intonations, grimaces, emotional reactions) that provide a clearer framework for evaluating the meaning of these statements.

Even if patients are provided with accurate probabilistic information there may be great difficulties dealing with the uncertainty associated with evaluating probabilities and applying them to personal behavior. We tend to deny that we are as personally vulnerable as the general population when we engage in hazardous but personally controlled risky behaviors such as flying or skiing (Slovic, Fischhoff and Lichtenstein, 1986). To avoid uncertainty we may cognitively reinterpret objective risk data into more predictable categories of occurrences. For example, small but unavoidable risks (1 chance in 1,000,000) may be treated as if they do not exist. A large risk (50 percent chance) may be recoded by the patient as a fait accompli. Moderate risks (such as a five percent chance) that cannot be placed in either category may be most alarming because it cannot be easily recoded, producing the greatest uncertainty (Epstein and Clark, 1970).

Recall biases

To make a decision, patients must recall pertinent information bearing on the decision and then evaluate those factors. However, as stated in Chapter 4, not all the information bearing upon the decision is "available" in memory. Only the most vivid and salient information is likely to be recalled. Pallid statistical data based upon a large number of experiences may be disregarded in lieu of a more vivid personal experience with one case (Borgidia and Nisbett, 1977). In addition, negative information may be more distinct than positive information and more easily recalled. A patient who knows of one person having had a negative experience with a therapy may fail to remember reading a favorable report.

As an expert, the advice of the physician is justifiably seen as important for recall. However, certain features of the medical encounter also favor the physician's advice for reasons unrelated to the doctor's expertise. The physician and the medical staff are both the providers of information and the seekers of decisions from the patient. There are several memory retrieval cues that favor recall of physician provided information rather than other relevant information stored in the patient's memory. The recency of the physician provided information makes that memory trace more retrievable. Even if the patient returns to the doctor's office and provides the decision on a revisit, the memory trace for the originally provided information is more easily activated because situational cues increase recallability (c.f., state dependent learning).

Weighing and evaluation bias

Evaluating relevant attributes presents a highly personal problem for most patients; which of the possible evaluation criteria are most important and how much should they be considered? Due to lack of experience, the patient simply may not know how to evaluate the criteria. In this instance the patient is reliant upon the doctor, becoming a passive participant in the decision making process. Many patients may fall into this category and many doctors, responding to perceived patient preferences, assume that their role extends to making decisions for patient.

Patients who wish to participate in the decision making process but are unfamiliar with the criteria are also reliant on the doctor's judgment (Povar, Mantell and Morris, 1984). The patient may inappropriately focus on certain criteria simply because they are unfamiliar with the more pertinent criteria and cannot understand their implications.

For the most part, the criteria that should be considered most fully are those that have direct bearings on short term goals and long term values that underlie those goals. We have discussed how framing effects influence the selection of goals. In addition, long term values, and in particular values related to taking risks, may also influence the evaluation of therapeutic criteria.

Patients face conflicting values when choosing among their options. Not only are values relating to health and illness brought to bear, but so are values concerning trust in the doctor, personal control, self-worth, and the willingness to take risks. Research on the "risky-shift" suggests that following group discussion, individuals become more willing to take risks in certain situations (or less willing to take risks in other situations). One explanation for this shift in risk taking is that group discussion reinforces culturally held norms for or against risk taking (Rettig, 1966). In our culture, we presume a norm that reinforces risk taking to cure illness. The physician who introduces therapeutic options to the patient may also communicate certain risk taking norms to the patient. Doctors may differ in the extent that they hold norms for risk taking. If patients are informed about their options by a surgeon who is inclined to take risks, patients may be more likely to have a risk taking norm communicated. If a more conservative, risk-adverse family physician communicates the therapeutic options, norms against taking risks may be communicated.

Motivation to make decisions

The editing and evaluation stages of decision making postulated under prospect theory suggest a cognitive basis for decisions and fail to take into account motivations to make decisions. People vary across situations in their willingness and ability to actively engage in decision making. The perceived role of the patient vis-a-vis the doctor dictates the patient's willingness to participate in decision making. Furthermore, how the patient perceives situational elements and appraises the risks of the disease and its treatment influences the decision making sequence.

Janis and Mann (1977) have proposed a flow-chart model of how health care decisions involving stress or conflict stemming from perceived impending danger influences decision making. According to their model, if the patient perceives that no risk is involved, no decisions or consequent behavior is stimulated. With asymptomatic diseases or dangerous lifestyles, unless cued by an external source the patient may not perceive any threat, so the decision making sequence is never initiated. With certain therapies, patients may be unaware that the treatment produces risks or they may believe that the physician would inform them of significant risks and there is no need to search for additional information. For example, patients taking Accutane, a drug used to treat severe acne, may simply assume that any drug to treat acne must be relatively innocuous. In reality, the drug causes birth defects if taken during pregnancy. Since patients did not perceive a threat, they did not initiate any information search or decision making processes.

If the patient perceives a threat, but the physician provides acceptable protective action, the model predicts that patients will simply follow the advice without becoming involved in appraising the treatment. In this instance the patient is totally passive and simply accepts what the physician suggests. The patient is unaware of the risks of the proposed treatment or the risks and benefits of the alternatives. The model does not assume that risk information is sought for anticipatory coping. If patients do not believe that there is an effective treatment for their condition, they may lose hope and avoid any role in decision making. They may defensively avoid seeking information about their condition or its treatment. Thus, the Janis and Mann (1977) model suggests that thoughtful decisions are likely only when patients are motivated by some threat and they perceive some hope for a reasonable outcome from their treatment.

A more recent model of "precaution adoption" developed by Weinstein (1988) suggests a number of stages leading to the decision to take protective action. Prior to deciding to take some precautionary behavior the patient would first have to become aware of the hazard, believe that the hazard is significant, and acknowledge that they are personally susceptible to the risks involved. This model suggests that active decision making occurs only if patients believe themselves to be personally at risk. The physician, by being overly reassuring about the course of an illness, stifles active decision making by communicating that the threat is not significant or that the patient is not personally at risk (Buchsbaum, 1986).

Patient Consent and Risk Acceptance

In the past decade there has been increased pressure on health professionals to inform patients about the risks of treatment. The doctrine of "informed consent" has fostered a revolution leading to the routine disclosure of risks for many medical treatments. Although the need for informed consent is generally accepted, there is much confusion and debate about the reasons why informed consent is necessary.

In a large scale review of the issues, the President's Commission for the Study of Ethical Problems in Medicine and Biomedical and Behavioral Research concluded that informed consent was shared decision making between provider and patient based on mutual respect and participation (Abram, 1982). From this perspective, we may view consent as simply providing the patient a greater role in the decision making process. However, it is unclear what form this role does or should take.

Patient's role

Engel, Blackwell and Miniard (1986) suggest that we may separate the role of families in the purchasing of products into five role categories: gatekeeper (initiator of thinking about the need for the product), influencer (offering opinions about selection criteria, weights, alternatives, etc.), decider (performing the editing and evaluation of the prospects), buyer (purchasing the product), and user (using the product). Applying this typology to health care therapeutics, we can see patient as the buyer and user of therapy. The patient may also be the initiator of the sequence for symptomatic problems and the doctor may be the initiator for asymptomatic conditions or when asking the patient to return for a visit. However, the role definition of influencer and decider are not clearly delineated. Does the doctor offer opinions and the patient decide or does the doctor recommend and the patient accept? These two perspectives have political and practical implications for control of the encounter between doctor and patient and serve as the basis for much debate about the ethics of medical care. Patients and doctors differ in their perspective on this issue (AAFP, 1987).

Zarin and Pauker (1984) have proposed a mathematical solution to the issue of decision making control. They suggest a formal model for splitting up the decision making process so that the physician and patient each concentrate on their areas of expertise. The doctor supplies information about therapeutic effects and the patient supplies information about the meaning of those effects. Under their proposal, the physician delineates all the relevant outcomes of alternative treatments. The patient supplies a value or utility for each outcome. Although conceptually engaging, in practice the arduous process of delineating outcomes and obtaining utilities in an unbiased fashion seems overwhelming. Furthermore, it is unclear what decision making strategy should be used (they propose a compensatory model free of physician influence; however, patients may prefer a lexicographic model or letting the physician decide).

Optimal decision making

Although the President's Commission viewed informed consent as a sharing of decision making between doctor and patient, Fischhoff (1985) has suggested that cognitive and institutional barriers prevent patients from being active decision makers. Further, from the patient's perspective, Fischhoff contends that the issue of the patient's role in decision making is not particularly germane. Informed consent serves the provider's need to assure that legal obligations are met. For the patient it is more important to assure that the best option is chosen.

For Fischhoff, optimal decision making, not shared decision making, should be the basis of informed consent. The provider's task in informed consent situations is threefold: to persuade the patient that the chosen option is more attractive than other options, to make sure the patient recognizes the virtues of the chosen option, and to assure the patient that the decision making process utilized is optimal and unbiased.

While Fischhoff's emphasis on the outcome of the decision making process improves the quality of care and optimizes choice among options, his analysis ignores some of the important process elements discussed in the President's Commission report. Both sharing and optimizing decision making are laudable goals. However, neither goal is particularly easy to achieve. Physicians are subject to the same biases as patients in their estimates of risk among various medical procedures (Christensen-Szalanski, Beck, Christensen-Szalanski and Kospell, 1983). How to achieve both goals in an ethically feasible manner remains theoretically important but practically difficult.

Physician and patient perspective

Perhaps the most objective manner of implementing informed consent is to base operations on what patients and health professionals view as the defining characteristics, facilitators, and barriers to consent. From a survey undertaken by the President's Commission, it is clear that the majority of physicians view informed consent as the disclosure of information to patients about their treatment (59%) and its risks (47%) (Abram, 1982). A smaller percentage of physicians view patient understanding of their treatment (34%) or its risks (23%) as part of informed consent. About one-fourth (26%) of the physicians surveyed viewed informed consent as soliciting patients' permission for treatment. Additional surveys indicate that most physicians view the outcome of informed consent as invariably negative, intruding on the physician-patient relationship, decreasing effective communications, curtailing freedom, and decreasing personalization (Taylor and Kelner, 1987). Thus, physicians generally view informed consent as merely informing patients about treatments and their risks. Given the perceived negative consequences of disclosure, most American physicians apparently feel legally compelled to disclose risks and suffer the negative consequences.

Patients' views of informed consent differ markedly from those of physicians. In another survey undertaken by the President's Commission, a substantial proportion of the general public believed that informed consent meant that the patient was informed about treatment (44%) and an equally large proportion said it meant that the patient agreed to the treatment proposed by the doctor (44%). Many of the patients who stated that informed consent meant agreeing to treatment added that this included letting doctors do whatever they believed best or necessary. A smaller percentage (19%) said that informed consent meant that patients make decisions about treatment. Still smaller numbers believed informed consent was patient understanding (11%) or that it was a form to sign (7%). Thus, from the patient's perspective, both being informed and exercising some control over the decision making process constituted informed consent. However, this control need not be explicit decision making authority. For many it meant tacit approval or agreeing to let the doctor exercise the doctor's best judgment.

Many patients express the desire to be informed about treatments and their risks, but are willing to let the doctor make decisions. Even if upsetting, most patients welcome accurate information about the effects of their treatment (Wallace, 1986). As discussed earlier, understanding the risks of treatment so that one can anticipate and cope with its outcomes appears to be a basic motive underlying the desire for risk information.

Assessing probabilities

From the patient's perspective, risk information may not be particularly helpful in making decisions about treatment. Most risks are expressed in probabilities. However, small probabilities cannot be easily translated into the binary outcomes that the patient faces (will this event occur or will it not occur). For extremely rare events, the patient may assume that the event will not occur and treat the prospects as if the risk is nonexistent. However, when the outcomes of treatment are severe, the patient may review the outcomes and make decisions based on perceived ability to cope with the worst case.

Beeson and Globus (1985) studied decision processes following genetic counseling. The genetic counseling protocols called for a structured set of decisions laid out in a formal decision tree for the patient. However, the authors found that many (54%) of the patients made decisions about their willingness to risk bearing an affected child prior to the counseling session. The decision making strategy used by these parents analyzed whether or not they could cope with bearing and raising a child with the genetic disease. Thus, rather than attempting to understand probabilities associated with the possible outcomes or make a judgment about the optimal decision formula, the question faced by these parents was "am I willing and able live with this outcome."

For patients, sharing or optimizing decisions may be less germane than assessing if one can or cannot cope with the worst case outcomes. Although some analysts have suggested that the patient "accepts" risks having been informed of their possibility, the concept of risk acceptance seems more conducive to societal or institutional views about risk, where the approval of new products for marketing involves making certain that the risk-benefit ratio for new products is superior to existing products already on the market (Lane and Hutchinson, 1987). It is difficult to conceive that patients "accept" risks. Rather, it appears that they want some control in determining whether or not they are willing to live with the ramifications of the risky procedure or event.

Risk perception

Rather than understanding probabilities, the issue facing patients is the perceived meaning of different forms of risk. Considerable research has focused on understanding the characteristics or dimensions underlying the perception of risk (c.f., Slovic, 1986; Covello, 1983; Bechtel and Bibera, 1983). Using a psychometric paradigm, Kraus and Slovic (1988) report research in which 18 risk characteristics were factor analyzed resulting in two factors. The first factor was "dreadedness." This factor was composed of several items measuring, for example, whether the risk faced was controllable by personal diligence, dreaded, globally catastrophic, fatal in its consequences, high risk to future generations, not easily reduced, and involuntarily undertaken. The second factor was the extent to which the risk was "unknown." It was composed of several items measuring, for example, if the effects of the risk were known to science and to the individual, delayed, and not observable.

Therapies differ in the extent to which their effects are perceived as both dreaded and unknown. In the Kraus and Slovic studies, some therapies were rated as not dreaded-known (Darvon, Valium, and antibiotics), others were dreaded-known (open-heart surgery, morphine, and barbiturates), others were not dreaded-unknown (aspirin, oral contraceptives, and x-rays), and still others were dreaded-unknown (laetrile, lasers). Generally, most therapies scored moderately along each of the two dimensions. The effects of therapies were less dreaded than more vivid societal risks (e.g., nerve gas, nuclear weapons, terrorism) but more dreaded than commonly used products (e.g., household appliances, power tools, hair dyes). On the known-unknown dimension, the risks of therapies were rated in between some more common or publicized products (e.g., alcoholic beverages, motor vehicles, handguns) and the less common or tested products (e.g., solar electric power, food irradiation).

This risk perception taxonomy suggests that the extent to which patients know and dread the risks they face are the major elements of risk perception. We postulate that familiarity with the negative outcomes should influence risk perception. If one believes the risks are known (at least to science), one may analyze this worst case and make a judgment about personal tolerance. However, if risks are unknown, there is little basis for inference about its outcomes and such an analysis is not possible. Examination of the dreadedness dimension suggests that the most dreaded risks are those involving major societal disasters (e.g., nuclear war) rather than personal outcomes. The therapies mentioned as most dreaded tended to be ones where the individuals would have difficulty personally identifying with using the treatment (e.g., laetrile, morphine, barbiturates).

This implies that educating people about risk outcomes (the negative effects of therapy and their meaning to the individual's life) should improve risk perception. Although subject to the same biases, experts tend to have more accurate perceptions of risk than lay persons (Christensen-Szalanski, Beck, Christensen-Szalanski and Kospell, 1983; Keown, Slovic and Lichtenstein, 1984). This may be due to their greater understanding of the outcomes of a wide range of risky treatments, permitting a fuller perspective in which individual risks may be placed.

Unfortunately, how to educate people about therapies to improve risk perception is not well understood. One approach that offers some promise is research that assesses the "mental models" people hold about disease, treatments, and their risks. By understanding how people conceive of therapies, we may correct misunderstandings and build upon existing knowledge and its organization in memory (Jungermann, Schutz and Thuring, 1988).

Lau, Bernard and Hartmen (1989) measured common sense representations of people who described a recent illness. They found five components of most recent illness cognitions: identity of the illness, time frames for the illness, consequences of the illness, attributions about the cause of the illness, and beliefs about curing the illness. Individuals differed in the extent to which their belief systems had full representations about each of these components. These representations led to differing orientations toward the illness. People with strong "identity" and "cure" orientations were more likely to report visiting a doctor when ill. This research suggests that public educational strategies that focus broadly on the disease may not be particularly helpful at prompting specific behaviors. Rather, an educational focus that provides information consistent with the desired orientation would be more likely to prompt the desired behavior. If we wish to prompt visits to the doctor, educating people about how to identify the illness and how it can be cured would be a more compelling strategy.

Risk Communication and Compliance

A third reason that risk information may be conveyed from health professional to patient is to persuade the patient to adopt a desirable behavior. Although one would assume that the patient, motivated to maintain or achieve a healthier state, would follow the doctor's instructions, large numbers of patients fail to follow instructions. Noncompliance rates of 30% to 50% are frequently reported in the literature (Sackett and Haynes, 1976; Haynes, 1985; Ley and Morris, 1984; Roth, 1987).

It is often assumed that patients fail to follow prescribed regimens because they do not understand instructions or do not have the physical or cognitive skills to do what is expected. It has also been postulated that barriers such as negative side effects or complex regimens cause noncompliance. However, Conrad's (1985) study of patients with epilepsy demonstrated that for many patients, noncompliance is motivated by deeper meanings. In his study, patients failed to take their medication because they wanted to exert control over their illness. They resented being dependent upon a medication and wished to express independence.

We must assume that a certain percentage of patients have strong reasons to avoid following their doctor's instructions. For these patients, not following the doctor's orders is a coping strategy that helps them adapt to or master their illness. Merely providing instructions to these patients will not necessarily promote the desired behavior. These individuals must be persuaded that the behavior suggested is important, that their current coping strategy is inappropriate, and that there may be severe consequences to failing to follow the doctor's orders. Finding meaningful persuasive arguments to convince patients about the necessity of doing what the doctor suggests is an important element in promoting healthier behavior. Risk communication, therefore, may be an important means of improving the rate of compliance with the doctor's orders.

Reasons underlying noncompliance

There are several conceptual models that have been advanced to explain reasons for lack of behavioral compliance (Leventhal and Cameron, 1987). Simple medical and behavioral conditioning perspectives fail to provide an adequate overview of factors that have been shown to influence compliance. Communication, health belief, and self-regulatory models provide a more thorough analysis of conditions leading to improved compliance. Each of these models posits the importance of perceptions and appraisal of threatening events and their impact. In general, the most effective health messages are those that increase the perceived value of health goals (avoiding or ameliorating illness) or the perceived likelihood that a prescribed behavior will reduce threats to health or achieve a desired goal.

The Health Belief Model organizes the relevant beliefs that patients hold about their illness or its treatment into four categories; beliefs about the severity of illness, patient susceptibility to illness, benefits from taking the prescribed action, and barriers to taking action (Becker and Maiman, 1975). In a recent review of 46 studies of the Health Belief Model, Janz and Becker (1984) found that beliefs about barriers to undertaking the prescribed behavior (89%) were most often predictive of compliance, followed by beliefs about susceptibility to the disease (81%), beliefs about benefits of the recommended action (78%), and lastly, beliefs about the severity of the disease (65%).

Given this construct and set of findings, it is no wonder that physicians are more inclined to withhold therapeutic risk information, as it may be perceived as a barrier to using the therapy. The risks of the illness, not the risks of treatment, are more likely to be the focus of communication. Furthermore, the benefits of treatment, rather than their risks, are more likely to be communicated. However, by their very nature, any intervention powerful enough to cure, treat, or prevent disease, will also have negative effects. As discussed earlier, for most treatments doctors phrase therapeutic risks in terms of directions for use, so that the therapy will be utilized correctly with the least risk possible.

Limiting treatment

Certain treatments may have severe negative consequences if overused. Physicians and, occasionally, societal institutions, are inclined to more straightforwardly convey risks of these treatments to persuade patients to limit use of the treatment. For example, a strong case can be made for convincing people to limit medication subject to abuse or addiction. Drugs that may be used illicitly, such as pain killers, anti-depressants, and steroids, are often viewed as dangerous if used outside of an approved medical context. The difference between communicating risks for informed consent and for persuasive reasons is seen in two of the initial drugs for which the Food and Drug Administration required patient package inserts (PPIs).

In the late 1960's FDA first required that manufacturers of oral contraceptives include information in labeling directed to patients that informed patients about the risks of using the product. At that time, the most serious risk was the increased possibility of forming blood clots that could be fatal. It was presumed that patients needed to consent to undertaking this risk, as the individuals taking this medication were usually young, otherwise healthy women who were taking the medication to prevent a naturally occurring condition rather than treat an illness.

In the mid 1970's FDA required a PPI for oral estrogen drugs. These products were used by women to help them through the early stages of menopause. There was evidence that the drug was only effective during the initial phases of menopause and that prolonged usage increased the risk of certain forms of cancer. However, some women continued to take oral estrogens for several years. These women mistakenly believed that prolonged use of the product could retain softness of the skin. The PPI for this medication emphasized the risks of prolonged usage of estrogens in an effort to convince women to stop taking them after a few months.

The persuasive impact of risk messages, however, is problematic. Providing people with threatening, sometimes fear inducing, information can be effective, but often is frequently ineffective. Leventhal and Cameron (1987) concluded that the persuasive impact of threatening messages is short lived and does not necessarily lead to behavior change. In a recent review of the mass media communications literature, Job (1988) concluded that five conditions were necessary before fear operates as an effective persuasive device: (1) fear onset needs to precede the desired behavior, (2) the fear producing event needs to be perceived as a likely occurrence, (3) the specific desired behavior needs to be effectively communicated, (4) the level of fear produced should be controlled (offset) by the desired behavior, and (5) fear offset should reinforce the desired behavior, confirming its effectiveness.

Job's analysis suggests that messages intended to reduce the use of a treatment will only be successful if several conditions are met. First, patients must believe that their action (stopping the treatment) will alleviate the threat. For example, if patients taking oral estrogens believe that they have used the product for such a long time that their risk of getting cancer will not be reduced by stopping the therapy, there is no incentive to stop using estrogens. Secondly, the level of fear produced by prolonging the treatment must be adjusted to match the fear of the disease. For the estrogen patient, the fear of the embarrassing and discomforting symptoms of menopause immediately returning must be reduced, or the fear of cancer caused by estrogens must be increased, if the patient is to be persuaded to stop the regimen. Thirdly, any external event that increases the salience of cancer increases the persuasive impact of the therapy reduction message. If a friend gets cancer or if a vivid story appears on television, then the threat of the disease becomes increased. Similarly, if a vivid event occurs involving the negative elements of the disease or symptoms under treatment, then the fear level produced by the therapy may not be great enough to arouse motivations to stop treatment. Finally, reinforcements need to follow the suggested behavior. If the estrogen patient is shown that the feared symptoms of menopause do not return, or if the level of discomfort is not as great as expected, then the positive behavior may be reinforced and continued.

Although Job's analysis is helpful at analyzing the effectiveness of fear arousing messages, it fails to explain how individual patients may react to the risk messages. The diversity of findings in the literature regarding the effectiveness of fear appeals suggests there are complex communication and psychological processes undermining the processing and reaction to risk messages.

Maddux and Rogers (1983) provide a more cognitive based model of threat communications based on protection motivation theory. They presume that fear arousing communications are cognitively appraised along four dimensions: (1) the noxiousness or severity of the threatening event, (2) the probability of occurrence of the event, (3) the efficacy of the proposed coping response, and (4) perceptions about the degree to which the individual can effectively perform the required protective behaviors (self-efficacy). In their study, all four dimensions were related to adopting attitudes consistent with avoiding threatened actions.

Maddux and Rogers' analysis suggests that the effectiveness of a fear arousing message (e.g., facing addiction unless one gets off tranquilizers) depends not only on the fear produced by the consequences of not adopting the behavior, but also by patients' envisioning of their own ability to cope with the advocated behavior (e.g., a life without tranquilizers). Thus, skill training and confidence bolstering may be necessary to increase the impact of fear arousing messages.

The use of fear inducing messages to influence patient behavior is subject to ethical debate. Some justly question whether or not physicians or other health professionals should try to frighten patients into doing something that they may not otherwise choose to do. On the other hand, it may also be unethical for a physician to simply mention a negative outcome of overusing a treatment and not provide additional persuasive messages, in essence, abandoning the patient.

Eraker, Kirscht and Becker (1984) have suggested that provider responsibilities should be viewed in the broader context of the doctor-patient relationship. A mature discussion of risks and emotional responses may be developed over time as patients confront their beliefs and emotions about their disease and its treatment. The physician can help the patient develop cognitive and emotional coping responses that permit abandoning unnecessary and risky treatment. However, clear limits exist in the extent to which the physician can force a patient to engage in any behavior. Truthful and accurate communication is an ethical imperative.

Implications

The roles and responsibilities of patients in making judgments about treatment are not particularly well understood. In certain situations patients have the expertise to apply their own value system to analyze the desirability of one therapy compared to another. However, the complexity of risk and benefit information and the numerous biases in communicating risk information make unbiased decision making extremely difficult.

Trust in the physician is often viewed as the major criterion leading to a mutually beneficial selection of treatment, where both the patient and doctor remain satisfied with the choice and the process of selection. However, trust need not presume that the physician takes sole responsibility for making decisions (i.e., blind trust). Rather, trust encompasses empathy on the part of the physician to: (1) understand the important perspectives of the patient so that the patient's values may be incorporated in medical decisions and (2) communicate information that the patient needs to know to have a role in consenting or tacitly approving the selected treatment.

Trust must also extend in the opposite direction. Patients must be trusted with the information they need to undertake responsible roles. Even if the patient does not want to make a decision, the physician should not usurp the patient's responsibilities when ethics demand the patient's consent to treatment. The physician may need to permit the patient time to talk the decision over with others, learn more about the options from written sources, and rediscuss the issues at a later point.

The extent to which physicians project their values on the patient's situation is a continual matter of concern. If the patient engages in unhealthy behavior (continuing to use therapy in a harmful manner) the physician is ethically licensed to persuade the patient as fully as possible as long as risk information is honestly presented. However, the point at which persuasion ends and coercion begins is not easily perceived.

The relationship between doctor and patient is, therefore, a central issue in how judgments are made about medical treatments. Unfortunately, in an age of fragmented health care, the physician's ability to learn about the patient's value system is much diminished. Filling this void, patients may take more responsibility, not because they want to but because they have to. It would be a mistake to overly generalize these conclusions. For many patients, the doctor serves the classic role of a trusted family friend and advisor. Understanding the range of existing role relationships and constructing segmental models of patient decision making strategies are important research needs. In constructing these models, patient evaluations, as the "consumer" whose needs must be served, should be the major determinant of acceptance of the relationship. In the next chapter, we discuss how the outcomes of therapeutic decisions influence the consumer's view of medical care.

6
Effects of Risk Communication

In a perfect world, once physicians explain the benefits, risks, and directions for how to use a therapy, patients merely utilize the treatment, get better, and remain satisfied with the physician, the treatment, and their condition. Unfortunately, the world is far from perfect and the anticipation that problems may result from improper risk communication is a driving force that influences the flow of information between doctor and patient. In Boyle's (1983) survey, physicians were asked how frequently patients had problems with drug therapy. The great majority of physicians (95%) said that patients frequently or occasionally terminated taking medication prematurely, 89% said that patients frequently or occasionally neglected the proper dosage schedule, 72% said that patients frequently or occasionally suffered suggestion-induced side effects, and 69% said that patients frequently or occasionally resisted drug therapy.

In this chapter we examine the results of risk communications between doctor and patient. What are the pitfalls of risk communication and to what extent do anticipated negative outcomes occur? As shown in Table 6.1, following the doctor-patient interaction, a series of evaluative events and behavioral actions are undertaken that determine the ultimate success of the therapy. Following the doctor visit, the patient evaluates the visit and the doctor, and initially evaluates the therapy. At this point the patient may decide not to take the prescribed therapy. For example, the patient may consider the cost of a medication too high or may have similar medication at home. If the therapy is used, the patient may experience adverse effects which cause a modification or discontinuance of the regimen. The patient may misuse therapy by

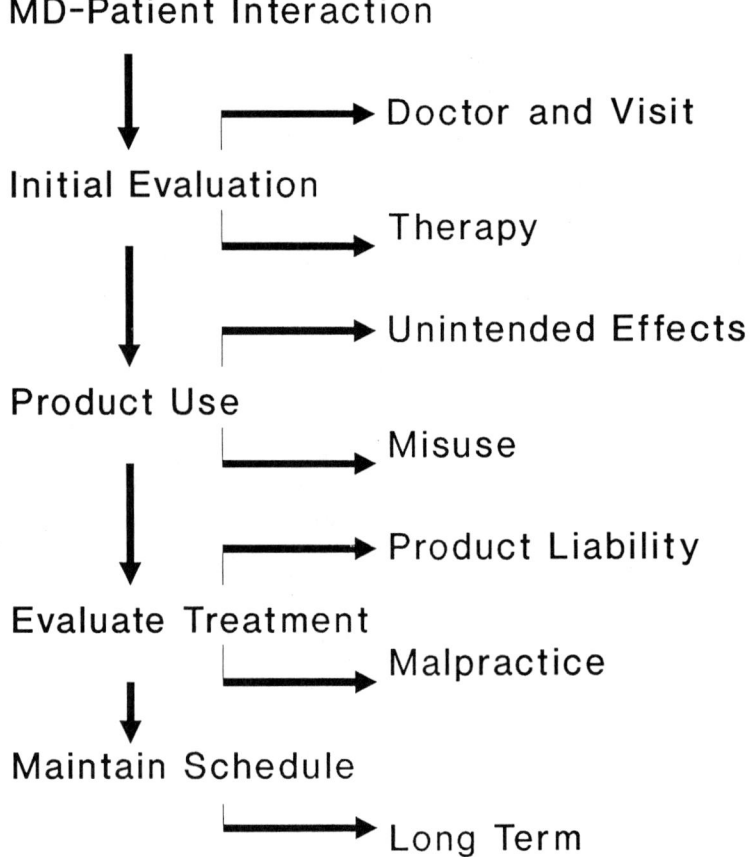

Table 6.1 Effects of Risk Communication

inappropriately increasing or decreasing the dosage level. Later during the regimen, adverse events or some other cue may cause the patient to reevaluate the treatment and make some judgment about overall satisfaction levels. Dissatisfaction may result in complaints and even a malpractice case being brought. If negative events do notoccur and/or the patient remains satisfied with the treatment, the patient may plan to continue with the treatment program. However, as we have noted before, maintenance of the dosage schedule is difficult to continue on an ongoing basis. For intentional or unintentional reasons, the patient may fail to follow the prescribed regimen.

Initial Doctor Visit

The doctor-patient relationship may be conceived as an ongoing, self-regulatory process or as a series of encounters with salient features that form the basis of an evaluation (Ware and Hays, 1988; Zastowny, Roughmann and Hengst, 1983; Mirowsky and Ross, 1983). Thus, we may ask patients about their views about the encounter, the relationship with a specific provider, or the general relationship between doctors and patients.

In a major review of 221 studies of patient satisfaction with doctors and treatment, Hall and Dorman (1988) found a direct linkage between information-giving and patient satisfaction. However, this overly general conclusion does not elucidate the important precursors of patient satisfaction. Hall and Dorman concluded that there is a "specificity effect" with patient satisfaction measurement. Patients report more satisfaction with recent and focused events or encounters than with generalized or ongoing relationships. Both cognitive and emotional bases for the specificity effect have been postulated. From a cognitive perspective, longer term evaluations foster the recall of salient, negative events. Negative events are likely to be vivid, distinctive, more easily recalled, and are more likely to become evaluated in the attitude formation task. Alternatively, from an emotional perspective, broader, long-term evaluations encompass a wider variety of needs that are left unfulfilled, resulting in more negative evaluations.

Numerous aspects of the encounter have been examined for their relationship to patient satisfaction. In a multidimensional scaling study, Smith, Falvo, McKillip and Pitz (1984) measured how patients viewed the ideal physician in terms of communication factors. They found a two dimensional solution best described their data. The ideal physician was rated as providing explanations (rather than rushing the appointment) and, secondly, paying attention to the patient rather than the nurse or the chart. Although this study suggests that paying attention to the patient and offering explanations leads to increased satisfaction, other studies have shown a more complicated relationship between physician behavior and patient evaluation. The patient's interpretation of the physician's attention and communication patterns rather than objective measures of the physician's behavior are essential to understand the necessary and sufficient conditions leading to patient satisfaction. For example, more humane physicians are more likely to have satisfied patients (Kallen and Stephenson, 1981), however, so are more proficient and task oriented physicians (Hall, Roter and Katz, 1987). Thus, there may be many complicated routes to satisfaction. It is necessary to understand how satisfaction evaluations are derived by patients and what function satisfaction serves in health care.

Expectations and outcomes

Linder-Pelz (1982) has defined patient satisfaction as a positive attitude about the health care they received. In her study, patient expectations were the single most significant predictor of patient satisfaction with treatment; the greater the discrepancy between expectations and observed occurrences the lower the satisfaction level.

Although the discrepancy between expectations and outcomes may serve as a general framework for predicting patient satisfaction with the doctor visit, the absolute expectation level is also important. Pascoe (1983) points out that patients in the Linder-Pelz study that had confirmed high expectations showed the greatest satisfaction levels whereas disconfirmed low expectation levels led to the greatest dissatisfaction.

Applying satisfaction measures from marketing models, Pescoe (1983) suggests satisfaction is a compensatory judgmental process and that its conceptualization and measurement requires attention to theoretical operations and assumptions that underlie its development. Specifically, it is important to understand what is expected (e.g., ideal outcomes, minimal standards, desired states, deserved treatments, normative values) and how expectations and occurrences are compared (e.g., contrasting with previous experience, assimilating inconsistencies to form a coherent evaluation, or within some latitude of acceptance that permits some deviation but not too much leeway).

Although many such operations are possible, Pescoe is unclear about how the expectation-occurrence matching process is made. All of the proposed derivations may occur under different circumstances. However, Pescoe suggests that there are two stages in the satisfaction evaluative process. As we discussed, there is an initial cognitively based evaluation. Secondly, an emotional reaction occurs based on the observed discrepancy.

Emotional reactions

The theoretical matching process between expectations and outcomes is useful for explaining the cognitive component of the satisfaction evaluation. Research based on norm theory (Kahneman and Miller, 1986) suggests that "emotional amplification" (i.e., the emotional reaction) is based upon an "envisioning" of how easily the observed occurrence could have matched an expected level. Norm theory suggests that expectations are not necessarily a priori expected performance levels. Rather, normative values, not necessarily a priori expected outcomes, can form the basis for an evaluation. The patient judges how easily it would have been for the physician to meet a normative level of performance. If patients discover, after a visit, that other doctors provide a service (e.g., telephone the patient the day after surgery to find out if there are any problems) that their doctor did not provide, the patient would become dissatisfied, even if the patient did not expect the service ahead of time.

Furthermore, emotional reactions may also be based upon the degree to which the patient perceives the physician as responsible for the low level of observed performance (c.f., Folkes, 1984). If the doctor is viewed as the cause of negative outcomes, the patient is more likely to be upset with the visit. There are three issues that guide this attribution process: (1) if the patient views that negative performance as unstable (sometimes the doctor meets my standards other times not), (2) if the failure has the physician as a "locus," or if the failure is due to some other factor (the doctor acted unreasonably when I requested the information, my request was not unreasonable) and, (3) if the outcomes are perceived as under the doctor's control (the doctor did not have any emergencies this morning and could have kept his appointments without keeping me waiting). Thus, cognitive appraisal is needed not only to judge the extent of the discrepancy but to direct emotional reactions to the correct target.

From this perspective, risk communications have several possible immediate influences on the evaluation of the doctor-patient interaction. If the patient does not expect any risk information about treatment, then disclosure of risks will violate expected norms. On the other hand, if risk information is expected but not delivered the physician may be perceived as not communicating necessary information. Whether expected or not, if the patient believes that risk information is usually provided to other patients (i.e., a stable outcome), that it is the physician's role to deliver the risk information (i.e., physician locus), and that the physician could have easily delivered it (i.e., physician control), then we would expect an emotionally upset patient.

In addition to providing risk information, giving patients greater control of risky outcomes appears to have emotional benefits. In a study of emotional reactions to surgery, Morris and Royle (1988) found that patients and spouses offered a choice of radiation or surgery as treatment for breast cancer had less negative anxiety and depression following the treatment compared to patients not offered the choice. Evidently, a greater role in therapeutic decision making and risk taking reduced emotional reactions to the treatment. At six months, differences between the choice and nonchoice groups was reduced; however, those not offered a choice still showed higher levels of anxiety and depression. The authors concluded that the choice of treatment reduced distress. However, they did not postulate about the psychological mechanisms underlying stress reduction.

Need fulfillment

We have earlier hypothesized that risk communication serves coping needs. Mastery and control are major needs that underlie the desire for risk information. However, other needs and coping styles may negate and even contraindicate the disclosure of risk information. Carver, Scheier and Weintraub (1989) have suggested that there are large individual differences in coping styles and strategies. Coping responses need to be applied to both the cognitive appraisal of risk and emotional reactions to the risks. In their review of the literature and subsequent evaluation, Carver, Scheier and Weintraub suggest fourteen different coping styles that may be adopted. Some of these styles include active coping and planning (taking direct action), concentrating on the action (putting aside other competing activities, restraining oneself from overreacting), seeking social support for both behavioral and emotional reasons, learning to accept and live with the problem, turning to religion or alcohol, actively denying the problem, or mentally or physically disengaging oneself from the problem.

Given this complex set of coping needs, it is no wonder that the same objective set of risk information may help some people cope and be of little value, or negative value, to others. Understanding coping strategies or helping patients find effective coping strategies requires active interaction with sensitive health professionals. Clearly, we need to have a greater understanding of what coping strategies patients use, how these strategies change over time, and how risk information serves their ever changing needs.

Initial therapy evaluation

In addition to evaluating the doctor and the visit, after the initial prescribing of treatment the patient either implicitly or explicitly forms an evaluation of the proposed treatment and decides whether or not to follow directions. Explicit evaluations are evident when patients obtain second opinions for surgical procedures. In an evaluation of a mandatory second opinion program, Rosenberg, Gorman, Snitzer, Herbst and Lynne (1989) found that emotional needs were served as well as informational ones. The respondents in their survey cited reassurance (59%) as the most common reaction to the second opinion. They also cited help in making the decision (49%) and having an opportunity to ask questions (29%) as other advantages to the mandatory program.

Implicit evaluations of therapy are evident by patient refusal to obtain prescribed therapy. Levy (1989) estimates that 14% of the prescriptions written are never filled. It is unclear if these prescriptions are for essential medications, if the patient is able to obtain the medicine from another source, or if the patient has some medicine left over from the last prescription taken. Unfortunately, with recent increases in prescription prices, it is probable that many people may not obtain ordered prescriptions because of their cost.

If patients are in tight financial straits, they may need to make a cost-effectiveness evaluation (is the treatment worth its costs) as well as a risk-benefit evaluation (are the benefits of treatment worth taking its possible risks). Providing risk information should most directly influence perceived risks. However, it may also influence perceptions of perceived benefits. For example, patients may perceive products that have certain risks to be more powerful or potent (c.f., Morris, Ruffner and Klinberg, 1985). In addition, risk information may also have influences on the cost-effectiveness evaluation of treatment. For example, patients may perceive the treatment as preventing them from working, thereby increasing the therapy's costs. If providing information about the risks of medication influences patients' desire to initiate therapy, simply not obtaining the prescription is a passive way to refuse treatment without confronting the doctor. Good data on how risk information influences prescription filling is difficult to find.

Product Use

Most patients obtain and start the regimen as proposed by the prescribing physician. Hopefully, the medication improves the patient's condition and is taken faithfully for its full course. However, for many patients the medication causes unintended side effects. In a recent study of the elderly and their medication, Cartwright and Smith (1988) found that 15% of respondents reported some symptoms or side effects after starting the regimen.

Suggestion induced side effects

One of the major concerns about providing people with risk information is that the number of side effects will increase because people are highly suggestible. Loftus and Fries (1979) have suggested that providing people with risk information can be "hazardous to their health" because of placebo induced side effects. We have seen that many doctors view suggestion induced side effects as occurring quite often in their practice (Boyle, 1983). Indeed, in a classic report by Pogge (1963), 23% of patients given placebos reported the occurrence of side effects.

However, in sick people, symptoms occur frequently that may or may not be due to taking medication. Even healthy people report spontaneous symptoms that could be considered side effects if they were taking medication. Reidenberg and Lowenthal (1968) interrogated healthy volunteers, not in treatment, and found that 81% reported some symptoms that, had they been taking some treatment, might have been considered a side effect.

In an effort to discern how the knowledge that one has taken a pill influences the reporting of side effects, Shapiro, Chassen, Morris and Frick (1974) gave patients a placebo tablet and asked them to report the occurrence of new symptoms after waiting in a quiet room for an hour. A second (control) group of patients were not given the placebo but asked to report on how their symptoms varied spontaneously after an hour. There was no statistical difference in the percentage of subjects who reported side effects in the placebo (61%) and control (64%) conditions. However, those who received the placebo were more likely to label their symptoms as primarily somatic (e.g., headache, burning eyes, stomach pain) whereas those in the control condition labeled their symptoms as primarily cognitive or affective (e.g., crying, upset, feeling sorry for self). Thus, people expect medicines to produce physical changes and label observed bodily state changes as such.

The suggestion that a medicine causes side effects influences how observed reactions are labeled, as drug effects or due to some other cause. In the Cartwright and Smith (1988) study, only 6% of the subjects reported no symptoms following the ingestion of medication. Evidently, people discriminate carefully between the medication and other explanations as the source of the symptom.

To provide a direct test of how risk information influences the occurrence and reporting of side effects, Morris and Kanouse (1982) provided a group of hypertensive patients with explicit information in the form of a brochure that listed the side effects of the medication they were taking. A control group was not provided the brochure. At the next revisit subjects who received the brochure were able to correctly name more of the side effects than control patients.

Also, at the revisit subjects were asked to report any new problems they experienced and whether or not they believed that the problems were caused by the medication. Seventeen health problems were specifically probed, some listed in the brochure as side effects. There was no statistical difference between the groups in the number of problems reported. A power analysis confirmed that there was small likelihood that the provision of the side effect information increased the number of problems experienced. However, there was a significant difference in the attribution of symptoms. Patients receiving the brochure were more likely to attribute experienced problems to the medication. Problems that were listed in the brochure were more likely to be attributed to the medication than problems that were not listed. However, even the unlisted problems were likely to be attributed to the medication for subjects who received the brochure, especially problems that were similar to the ones listed in the brochure.

Providing of side effect information promotes attribution effects rather than suggestion effects. If people view their therapy as a source of health problems they are more likely to discriminate side effects from other naturally occurring states. Patients who are informed about drug side effects may be better able to discriminate those effects and, therefore, deal with them more appropriately if they occur. For example, if a person perceives increased urination frequency as a side effect of a medicine, then that person can rearrange the dosage schedule to assure that the timing of the urination does not disrupt sleeping patterns or important occasions. Dodd (1984) has shown that it is important to include self-care instructional techniques along with information about the occurrence of side effects to assure that patients understand how to treat side effects if they do occur.

On the other hand, the data also suggest that people do not necessarily remember the precise names of side effects and label bodily state changes with those names. Rather, patients appear to remember some vague sense of the side effects that may occur and tend to attribute similar effects as side effects of the medicine. Thus, there is a possibility that nondrug effects could be attributed to the medicine. As the science of pharmacoepidemiology is imprecise, it is unlikely that scientists can necessarily correctly discriminate drug and nondrug effects. Perhaps, more importantly, we need to ask how the increased attribution of side effects to the medicine influences drug taking and health care. A recent study by Myers, Cairns and Singer (1987) suggests that informing patients about side effects increases the number of patients who drop out of treatment. In a multicenter study of drugs used to prevent angina, subjects in two of the centers were informed that the medication could increase the occurrence of gastrointestinal side effects, while at the third center subjects were told that the drugs were well tolerated by most patients. There was no difference between the centers in the number of serious gastrointestinal side effects experienced. However, the number of minor gastrointestinal side effects experienced at the two centers where patients were preinformed was increased relative to the third center. Also, more patients in the two centers dropped out of treatment because of these minor gastrointestinal symptoms.

If patients informed about the risks of treatment attribute observed symptoms to the medicine, the possibility that these attributions lead to discontinuation of treatment must be considered. Studies of patients' compliance with therapeutic regimens indicates that many patients who stop their medication cite side effects as the cause. In the Cartwright and Smith (1988) study, 40% of the people who stopped taking their medication cited the experience of side effects as the major reason for discontinuation. Dodd's (1983) research in which self-care information was provided along with the side effect profile suggests that it is important to provide patients with viable options for dealing with side effects.

Product misuse

Another problem of providing risk information is that fear about therapy may induce patients to misuse the product. For example, patients may underdose or fail to use an indicated product because of fear of long term side effects. Lee and Lipton's (1983) review indicates that "intelligent noncompliance" (the willful misuse of a product because of fears of ingesting excessive amounts) is a major reason for drug misuse among the elderly. Stephens, Haney and Underwood (1982) asked noncompliant patients why they did not follow the regimen. The most common reason given (by 49% of the respondents) was that they did not like to take medication.

Although fear of side effects and negative outcomes may be cited as a reason for underusing a product, there may be other uncited reasons. Risk information can serve to rationalize underlying motives. Medical philosophers have categorized numerous values underlying the use of medication (Veatch, 1980). Ethics based upon the avoidance of unnatural products or "if it makes you feel good it must be wrong" (pharmacological Calvinism) compels people to avoid taking medicine (Klerman, 1979). There are many "latent motives" underlying medication avoidance. This motive necessitates an objective external reason for not taking medication. The risk of side effects provides a manifest reason that justifies underuse.

Treatment Evaluation

In addition to evaluating the visit with the doctor and initially evaluating the therapy, patients also evaluate therapy after they begin the regimen. This evaluation is likely to be cued by an event such as the doctor or a friend asking how the treatment is working or simply noticing that the treatment is causing behavioral or bodily state changes. Noticing a positive change is likely to result in positive satisfaction ratings. Lack of change could lead to dissatisfaction, trepidation, or a "wait and see" evaluation.

Another event that causes evaluation is the occurrence of new symptoms, sometimes quite severe. If serious side effects do occur, the a priori provision of risk information has serious ramifications for how patients react physically, emotionally, and legally. If something "goes wrong," an attribution process is spurred and the patient must decide if the patient, the doctor, or the product is at fault. Wagener and Taylor (1986) examined attribution process of patients who had successful and failed renal transplant operations. Patients who had failed transplants tended to lessen their own perceived responsibility, diffusing responsibility for the decision. The authors propose that the diffusion of responsibility for the decision was a result of cognitive dissonance. Thus, if something goes wrong, patients are motivated to blame someone or something other than themselves for the failure. If the patient is dissatisfied but not seriously harmed, some complaining action may be initiated. If the patient is seriously harmed, however, product liability or malpractice cases may be initiated as a result of this attribution process.

As cited above, side effects of medical treatment are quite common. However, most of these side effects (such as fatigue, dizziness, and upset stomach) are transient and dissipate if the therapy is continued. For some people, these side effects may produce a hardship (fatigue can be a major problem for a truck driver). For others, the same side effect may be mild and merely a nuisance. How the individual reacts to these common side effects can vary greatly. Some may continue on the regimen and endure the side effects in light of the perceived benefits of the medication. Others may discontinue the regimen. Complaining behavior also varies, as some endure without complaining, while others complain to their friends, to the medical staff, or to the doctor directly.

More serious adverse reactions may cause the patient to seek additional medical help. In a recent review, Nolan and O'Malley (1988) found estimates of hospital inpatients suffering adverse drug reactions to range from 1.5% to 44% (with the largest study placing the estimate at 5.6%); for people applying for hospital outpatient treatment the estimates of problems caused by adverse drug reactions ranged from 2.2% to 50.6% (with the largest study placing the rate at 2.2%); and for hospital inpatient admission due to adverse drug reactions the estimates ranged from 2.9% to 7.9% (with the largest study placing the rate at 3.7%). Even with these relatively small percentages, the large number of hospital admissions for inpatient and outpatient treatment makes the absolute number of cases of serious iatrogenic disease enormous.

Although the number of product liability and malpractice cases has increased dramatically, a relatively small percentage of possible cases are brought to the legal system (Danzon, 1986). The way in which patients, their lawyers, and the courts apportion blame, and the impact of risk communications on this attribution process, is an important determinant of product liability and malpractice.

Product liability

Under product liability law, the manufacturer of a product is strictly liable for all injuries caused by defects in the product even if all possible care is used in the manufacture of the product. A defect may be due to a deviation from the design of the product (construction defect), from a product design that causes unnecessary risks (design defect), or from inadequate warnings (warning defect). With medical products, even if all possible care is used in the design and manufacture of the products, the product may still pose risks. However, the benefits of the product outweigh its risks. These products are, therefore, "unavoidably unsafe." Thus, medical products may knowingly pose certain risks but are not necessarily defective or unreasonably dangerous if directions for use and warning information are provided (c.f., Gilhooley, 1986).

The purpose of product liability law is to protect the consumer from exposure to unnecessary or unreasonable risks. As the risks of many medical products are known to science, the case for informing the consumer is quite strong. Nevertheless, the courts have maintained that the physician serves as a "learned intermediary" between the manufacturer and the patient. The duty of the manufacturer is to warn the physician and the physician's obligation is to protect the consumer.

The learned intermediary defense has withstood the assault of many law suits against medical product manufacturers where patients have sought direct warnings from the manufacturer. In early cases, the courts maintained that risk information would serve no useful purpose for the patient as the patient could not evaluate the information. Even if the patient objected to using a drug, the drug may still be necessary to save the patient's life (Rheingold, 1964). More recent cases have given more autonomy to patients for understanding risk information. However, the rulings have maintained that since the physician makes the decision about treatment, the physician must decide what facts should be told to the patient. The provision of risk information directly to the patient could interfere with the doctor-patient relationship and is, therefore, viewed as legally unnecessary.

There have been a few exceptions to the learned intermediary defense. Vaccines and mass immunizations have been found to lie outside the learned intermediary defense. As patients do not routinely see the doctor to obtain this therapy, there is no opportunity for the doctor to diagnose, choose a treatment, and inform the patient. In these cases, manufacturers have been held liable for not distributing warnings about the treatment. However, the absence of a physician during routine medical treatment has not increased product liability. For example, in a case where a patient was taking a glaucoma drug for many years without the constant supervision of the medical staff, and the patient suffered kidney stones, the courts held that the manufacturer was not liable for providing direct patient warnings. The physician still prescribed the drug initially (Gilhooley, 1986).

A second exemption to the learned intermediary defense involves oral contraceptives. The courts have viewed oral contraceptives as having peculiar characteristics. As discussed earlier, patients who use oral contraceptives are actively involved in making decisions about their use. Since the patient actively makes decisions about their use, the courts have held that oral communication between doctors and patients is insufficient and that direct communication of the product's risks from the manufacturer is essential. The fact that the federal government has required patient package inserts for oral contraceptives reinforces the court's conclusions.

Recent cases in Michigan and Massachusetts have bolstered the warning messages required for oral contraceptives. The Michigan court has held that the patient could reasonably refuse to take oral contraceptives without rejecting life threatening treatment. Furthermore, in the case of Stephens v. G. D. Searle & Co. the court held that since the manufacturer had directed publicity at consumers, the company had an obligation to disclose risks directly to consumers.

In Massachusetts, the case of MacDonald v. Ortho Pharmaceutical Corp. has added to the scope of warnings necessary for the manufacturer to divulge. The court found that the manufacturer had failed to provide adequate warnings. Although the manufacturer's brochure had divulged the fact that oral contraceptives could cause potentially fatal blood clots, the brochure did not mention that the drug could cause strokes. Having suffered a stroke and paralysis, MacDonald maintained, and the court upheld, that there are fates worse than death. If the prospect of paralysis had been made known, she would not have taken the medicine. Thus, manufacturers have a duty to disclose information that may be dispositive to a decision about whether or not to take the risk of using an inherently unsafe product.

Medical malpractice

The learned intermediary defense essentially sets up the doctor for taking the brunt of legal offenses. Although a plaintiff attorney may wish to sue the party that has the "deepest pockets" in a failure to warn case, the manufacturer carefully and systematically issues warnings to health professionals. Except in cases where the plaintiff can show that the manufacturer withheld information or knowingly marketed a product without disclosing necessary risks, the manufacturer is usually protected from direct liability. Doctors, and the hospitals in which they perform their duties, then become the focus of legal liability cases. To a much lesser extent pharmacists also face legal liability (Brushwood and Simonsmeier, 1986).

While a negative event following therapy is the cue for initiating a suit, few patients follow through with suing their doctor.

In a 1982 survey, 13% of patients stated that they had at one time considered suing a doctor. This figure was up from 8% when the same question was asked in a 1976 survey (Brown, 1983). However, less than one percent of patients bring law suits.

In an analysis of the reasons why patients sue their doctors, Avery (1986) asked the attorneys at an insurance company to identify the single most important reason behind the filing and participation in medical malpractice cases that the insurance company handled in the past year. The attorneys rated physician communications (failure to disclose risks and failure of the doctor to respond to a request for presence) and physician attitude (hurried, air of superiority, appearing cold and indifferent) as the two major reasons for malpractice law suits (each reason accounted for 35% of the lawsuits). Other reasons cited were: financial incentives (10%), media play about malpractice (7.5%), disparagement of the physician (7.5%), and unrealistic expectations (5%).

In a scenario study of consumer reactions to malpractice situations, Brown and Swartz (1984) studied demographic and attitude correlates of the propensity to enter into a malpractice case. Younger male patients signified a greater propensity to sue the physician in a malpractice case. Those who signified they were more likely to sue also indicated that they had a stronger desire for information about treatments, and believed doctors charged too much, but wished that the doctor spent more time with them explaining treatments.

Brown and Swartz (1984) also surveyed consumers and physicians about possible solutions to the malpractice problem. Physicians favored institutional solutions to the malpractice crisis. They strongly endorsed laws that would: (1) place caps on malpractice claims and lawyer fees or (2) force cases to go before a medical board. Consumers were somewhat in favor of these solutions; however, they were more in favor of greater time being spent by the doctor explaining possible problems. Spending more time with the patient was the only solution in which physicians and patients did not differ in the extent to which both groups favored the solution.

Inadequate communication is the most frequently suggested cause and increased communication the most desired solution to malpractice cases. However, it is unclear what form this increased communication should take. Simply talking more does not necessarily improve consumer satisfaction and may not improve protection against litigation. Weisman, Teitelbaum and Morlock (1988) found that physician attitudes about communication were generally unrelated to the frequency of malpractice claims and threats against obstetricians and gynecologists, except for the counterintuitive finding that physicians who had a more positive attitude about patients seeing their medical records were more likely to have been named defendants in a lawsuit (perhaps the attitude resulted from the case).

Examination of the medical practice management literature, in which doctors discuss anecdotal cases and propose solutions to malpractice problems, suggests that doctors view malpractice as a problem of socio-emotional communications rather than an instance of professional incompetence. Prather (1989) suggests that physicians equalize the level of communication, asking patients for their opinions, never promise more than a treatment can deliver, explain reasons for suggested treatment, and allow patients and their family time to vent their anger if a treatment goes wrong. O'Donnell (1986) suggests that it may be necessary to explain to patients what diagnostic solutions can be ruled out or actively considered so that the patient does not lose confidence in the physician (e.g., "you do not have cancer" or "you may have Alzheimers disease"). However, he also suggests that this information may unnecessarily worry some patients.

Still other literature directed to physicians suggests how doctors can spot patients who are likely to sue (Brown, 1983). Doctor-shoppers, noncompliers, flatterers, consumerists, and unhappy patients are viewed as more likely to sue. In these cases, the patient is viewed as the locus of the suit rather than an incompetent doctor. Incompetent doctors are viewed as "rogues", unethical and uncaring (Holoweiko, 1989).

In this atmosphere of malpractice threats, doctors should be more willing to disclose risk information in an effort to avoid unpleasant surprises. However, risk information should be carefully phrased to circumvent upsetting patients. A greater sharing of physician fears and uncertainties may tend to equalize the role relationship between doctor and patient, increase the patient's sense of control, and reduce patient uncertainty by narrowing down options. However, it may also increase patient fears and anxiety about the threats faced by the illness and its treatment (Gutheil, Burszajn and Brodsky, 1984). Furthermore, as Wagener and Taylor's (1986) study indicates, patients may be motivated to avoid accepting responsibility if something goes wrong. Suchman and Matthews (1988) have suggested that the essence of the doctor-patient relationship is the degree to which the doctor and patient become "connected" in the sharing of meaning and emotion. Special moments of sharing between doctor and patient, termed "connexional experiences," form the basis for this relationship.

For physicians, it would seem to be important to understand the coping response being used by patients and offer information and support that helps the patient cope with their illness. Unfortunately, the coping response chosen by the patient may not be the most adaptive or may not be in concert with legal obligations of the physician. For example, if the patient is actively denying the treatment of the illness, the physician may still be obligated to discuss the illness and its treatment. The saving grace in these circumstances may be the long term relationship between doctor and patient. It may be possible for the doctor to disclose partial risk information at a certain time and after the patient adjusts to that information, disclose additional risks. A long term relationship, where risks are disclosed in a context that permits the patient to adjust and cope with the new risks in a supportive surrounding offers a great advantage in communication acceptance.

Maintaining Treatment

The last stage, and ultimate goal, of evaluation following the doctor-patient interaction is the successful maintenance of the scheduled regimen. The factors that influence initial evaluation and decisions to initiate a treatment regimen may be quite different from the factors that facilitate or inhibit long term maintenance of the dosage schedule. As the population has aged, therapies have become more chronically oriented. The need for patients to actively monitor their treatment on a long term basis has continued to increase and greater emphasis has been placed on maintenance of long term dosage schedules. Models that focus on maintaining behaviors rather than decision making have helped elucidate factors that influence these long-term actions.

Green, Kreuter, Deeds and Partridge (1980) have proposed a health education model based on the voluntary adoption of health promoting behaviors. The PRECEDE model is based upon an educational diagnosis of the patient's predisposing (attitude and value orientation), enabling (resource availability), and reinforcing (response of other personnel) factors that maintain health promoting behaviors.

The PRECEDE model proposes a variety of educational interventions targeted to achieve particular goals. For example, to increase awareness, one may start with cheaper audiovisual communication strategies and follow up with more expensive group lecture and discussion for patients who need additional interventions. The PRECEDE model provides a useful framework for organizing educational interventions. However, the model is fairly general, cutting across many types of health care problems. A more in depth understanding of individual problems must precede the application of the PRECEDE model.

It is clear that certain behaviors are more easily maintained than others. Weinstein (1988) has suggested that the degree of effort necessary to maintain certain behaviors will vary with the particular behavior. For example, simple switch behaviors (substituting Tylenol for aspirin for a child with flu or chicken pox to reduce the risk of Reyes Syndrome) are easily maintained. There is no difference in effort in using one product over another.

However, other behaviors are more difficult to maintain. Once diagnosed as a diabetic, individuals need to give themselves injections every day. There may be an initial adjustment period during which people must not only learn to perform the behaviors necessary to treat themselves, but how to incorporate these behaviors into daily activities. Once incorporated into daily routines, the effort necessary to maintain the behavior is reduced, but still requires some effort and planning for it to be maintained.

A more common example is the adoption of simple behaviors, such as taking medication every day or several times a day. There is no great effort initiating the regimen (assuming that the patient decides to start it). Over time, the effort to maintain the treatment should be reduced as the behavior becomes incorporated into the patient's schedule. However, other situations (while away from home) and stress (emotional reactions to other factors) may inhibit maintenance of the schedule. Learned behaviors may not be performed if the environment in which the behavior is learned is substantively different from the environment in which the behavior is to be performed.

If a behavior is performed on a routine basis, with minimal thought and effort, the behavior may become automatic (Alba and Hutchinson, 1987). For example, brushing one's teeth every morning to start the day may become automatic. We do not necessarily think about performing the behavior, we simply engage in the response. Unfortunately, automatic behavior builds up very slowly, and only with a great deal of overlearning of very specific skills. It is possible that certain risk adaptive behaviors may become automatic. An individual who is a diabetic from childhood may view the morning injection of insulin as automatic.

To encourage long term maintenance, a number of strategies have been suggested. These strategies seek to structure an environment in which learned behaviors will be performed. Green, Mullen and Stainbrook (1985) have suggested five strategies for reducing drug dosage scheduling errors among elderly patients. The strategies that they propose focus on: (1) relevance - the suggestions given to the patient should be relevant to educational level and lifestyle (it makes no sense to tell someone to read about a drug if the individual is illiterate); (2) individualization - the proposed treatment must fit in with the individual's lifestyle (there is little sense in telling a patient to take a drug three times a day after every meal if the individual snacks all day and does not eat full meals); (3) feedback - providing patients with information on how well they are performing should increase their ability to maintain the schedule (records showing blood pressure levels over time may provide feedback to the individual about how well they are maintaining a drug regimen); (4) reinforcement - encouragement to maintain the schedule can help long term health behavior change (using other family members to provide social support can be an effective mechanism for improving maintenance of dosage schedules); and (5) facilitation - providing physical cues that help maintain the treatment can aid in long term strategies (using unit dosing packages or reminder buzzers can help prompt the desired behavior).

Long term maintenance of behavior appears to be a difficult goal to achieve. All these strategies, or some combination of them, are necessary for achieving long term maintenance. Simple information giving does not appear to be a sufficient condition for achieving long term maintenance (Morris and Halperin, 1979). Rather, behavioral intervention, in addition to information giving, appears necessary. These interventions may be as complex as contracting with other family members for social support strategies or as simple as sending out reminder post cards to provide cues for prompting desired behavior (Mayer and Frederiksen, 1986)

Green, Mullen and Friedman (1986) have suggested that the health professional "triage" the patient depending upon an educational diagnosis. Thus, patient education and therapy maintaining interventions could be applied in a more selective fashion. An individualized intervention could then be used to tailor the educational strategy for the individual. Hatcher, Green, Levine and Flagle (1986) have devised and adapted such triaging "rules" for hypertensive patients and shown improvements for these educational interventions.

There may already be some natural triaging that goes on in every day practice as physicians and their staff develop strategies to improve the maintenance of health care behaviors. In future years we may be able to develop a better understanding of how patients' "aptitude" matches proposed treatments. Early work with matching patient "aptitude" with specific treatments has shown disappointing results (Dance and Neufeld, 1988).

One possible way of improving the match between patient aptitude and the selected intervention is to provide patients with a greater choice in their selection of educational and behavioral strategies to improve health maintenance behaviors. Morris and

Royce (1988) found emotional benefits from providing patients with a greater choice in selecting treatments. Segmenting patients into homogeneous groups according to responsivity to maintenance strategies may be a first step in such a choice process. There may be some increased patient motivation to maintaining a behavior if the patient views themselves to be the initiator of the action. However, more specific data testing this concept is needed before more fully developed recommendations can be made.

Implications

After the patient visits the doctor the therapy begins. Risk communication is liable to influence early evaluations in several ways. If adverse reactions are unexpected, but do occur, patients may become cognitively and emotionally dissatisfied, not only because the product did not perform as expected, but because they were not told about the risks. It is difficult to emotionally separate evaluation of the therapy and evaluation of the doctor who prescribed the treatment. The degree to which patients view the doctor as making the decision without their consent or withholding information that could have easily been provided influences the attribution and evaluation process.

For the doctor, the legal obligation to inform the patient about risks and the emotional obligation to protect the patient from harm appears to be in conflict. Perhaps some stimuli that cue the discussion of therapeutic risks at a revisit would help the patient receive risk information. Unfortunately, the cue that currently serves to stimulate discussion is the occurrence of side effects, which may itself lead to negative evaluations, therapeutic discontinuation, or a law suit.

Although maintaining treatment is a laudable goal, it is more often the goal of the health professional than the patient. Pharmacological Calvinism may inhibit patients from valuing long term therapy maintenance. Successful maintenance is most likely when patients and physicians agree on the value of the treatment (Starfield, Wray, Hess, Gross, Birk and Lugoff, 1981). Physicians need to assure that patients understand the importance of their treatment. With this broader view of the importance of treatment, risk information can be evaluated from a more sensible perspective.

It is unrealistic to place the burden for teaching the patient solely on the doctor's shoulders. The physician may be more pragmatically viewed as managing the patient's treatment and education. Perhaps educational messages, along with risk disclosures, should come from the doctor's staff or some other health professional. Patient support groups may also be helpful at providing information relating to experienced therapeutic risks. In the next chapter we examine two nonpersonal means of providing therapeutic risk information to patients.

7
Mass Media Risk Communication

We have examined the communication of risk information primarily as it flows from health professional to patient. Interpersonal relationships modify risk communication, changing meanings and interpretations, and understanding these relationships is essential to understanding risk communication. However, patients receive risk information from other non-personal sources as well. The health education movement has fostered the growth of numerous print and audio-visual patient education materials (Green, Kreuter, Deeds and Partridge, 1980).

Patient education materials focus on achieving behavioral change, not communicating therapeutic risks. Rather, product risks have been delivered via warning labels that accompany certain products in public commerce or are incorporated as part of the advertising to assure that promotional materials are not misleading.

In this chapter we will examine the communication of therapeutic risks via these two mass media channels. First, we will explore historical developments and research evaluations of patient package inserts (PPIs) that accompany certain medications as part of their required labeling. Secondly, we will examine the societal factors promoting and hindering the communication of risk information disclosed in television advertising for prescription drugs (direct to consumer advertising of prescription medication (DTCA)). Unlike most advertising, prescription drug promotion is regulated under the Food, Drug and Cosmetic Act, which requires the disclosure of product risks within promotional materials. With pharmaceutical companies becoming interested in DTCA, incorporating risk disclosures in prescription drug advertisements is becoming an important public policy issue.

Historical Development of PPIs

To comply with the requirements of the Federal Food, Drug and Cosmetic Act, prescription drug manufacturers or repackers must include a copy of the official labeling, or "package insert," with each package they deliver. In the United States, pharmaceutics are usually packaged in bulk containers, which pharmacists use to fill individualized prescription orders. The pharmacist replaces the official labeling with a brief set of directions typed on a small label affixed to the container dispensed to the patient.

In the late 1960's, the Food and Drug Administration (FDA) departed from this usual practice on a few occasions and required manufacturers to include a PPI in addition to the package insert written for the health professional. We can examine the development of PPIs as progressing through four distinct phases of increasing and then decreasing interest as FDA first flirted, became infatuated, had a stormy break-up, and now has a cool, mature relationship with PPIs (Morris, 1989). While interest in the United States has waned, the European Economic Community has become quite interested in PPIs and intends to require them for distribution with prescription drugs as of 1992 (Sauer, 1989).

Phase one - the flirtation

The first product to have a required PPI was isoproterenol inhalators. It was found that these inhalators, intended to increase air passage flow, paradoxically could decrease air flow if overused. Given the self-administered nature of these preparations for attacks of bronchial asthma, a brief, two sentence warning was required informing patients not to exceed the prescribed dose.

In the early 1970's, FDA required a PPI for oral contraceptives. As mentioned earlier, the rationale for the oral contraceptive PPI was one of "patient consent." The accumulating evidence of thromboembolic disorders associated with the use of oral contraceptives, along with the elective nature of the pill and the availability of other means of contraception necessitated that patients be fully informed about the risks of using the pill. This would enable patients to participate more fully in the choice of birth control mechanisms. Initially, FDA required an abbreviated warning message attached to the package distributed to patients. The abbreviated warning informed patients that the continued supervision of a physician was necessary, that the drug caused serious side effects (especially blood clots), and that a longer brochure was available from their doctor. The brochure was a minimum of 14 paragraphs long (manufacturers were free to add additional material) and was intended to be distributed voluntarily by physicians to requesting patients.

The original content and distribution method for the oral contraceptive PPI was changed in the late 1970's as additional risks of using the pill became known and after an evaluation of PPI effectiveness (Morris, Mazis and Gordon, 1977). Both the abbreviated PPI and the brochure were lengthened to incorporate additional risk information and distribution of the brochure was switched from doctor to pharmacist.

In addition to the isoproterenol inhalators and oral contraceptives, in the late 1970's PPIs were required for oral estrogen products and progestins to assure that patients would obtain written warnings about the risks of using these products. Unlike the original two products, however, PPIs for these products were not prepackaged by the manufacturer. The pharmacist was required to store and distribute a separate instruction sheet. As one might have expected, an evaluation of the estrogen PPI found that only 39% of the pharmacists spontaneously delivered the PPI to individuals obtaining a prescription. However, 89% of individuals obtaining prescription orders were able to receive one if they requested it (Morris, Myers, Gibbs and Lao, 1980). FDA's conclusion at that time was that distribution rates would improve if dispensing PPIs became more routine.

Phase two - infatuation

At the same time that FDA was issuing regulations for individual PPIs for estrogens and progestins, it also investigated the desirability of broader scale implementation. Two strong social forces, consumerism and patient education, formed a climate conducive to PPI development.

The consumerism movement fostering PPI development was spearheaded by a petition issued by a consortium of consumer interest groups. They argued that PPIs were required to fulfill the consumer's right to know about prescription drugs. The petition reviewed evidence that verbally supplied information from the physician was frequently inadequate and was easily forgotten if provided. Given the hazardous potential for prescription drugs, the petitioners believed that written information providing instructions and precautions was needed for a majority of prescription medication (Morris, 1977).

About this time, spawned by public interest in reducing the incidence in hypertension, a great deal of publicity was generated by the broad scale problem of patients' lack of adherence with prescription medication regimens. Evidence was accumulating that communication failure was partly responsible for the problem of noncompliance. Additional literature indicated that written information could improve patient knowledge and schedule adherence for short term (antibiotic) regimens (Morris and Halperin, 1979; Brim, 1979). For longer term regimens, written information was viewed as part of a larger intervention needed to improve compliance rates.

To develop a PPI program, FDA initiated the Patient Labeling Project in 1974 to solicit advice from constituencies affected by PPIs, conduct research and evaluation studies, and design a PPI implementation plan. FDA solicited advice through both in-person meetings and in writing. Throughout the mid and late 1970's, FDA conducted small meetings, national symposia, and public hearings.

Consumer advocacy groups supported the program and advised that FDA proceed as rapidly as possible towards implementing requirements. At first, most health professionals were supportive of the problem of patient education but were skeptical that PPIs were a viable solution. As FDA further developed the program and issued plans for its implementation, polite skepticism turned to vehement resistance. Health professional associations became almost uniformly opposed to PPIs. Rather than define the PPI issue as an intervention aimed at the problem of patient education, health professional associations came to see it as an issue of too much government regulation.

From a research standpoint, FDA initiated studies to address three issues: (1) What information do patients need to know about their prescribed medication?, (2) How should the information be communicated? (i.e., the form and content of the PPI), and (3) What effects might we expect?

Surveys indicated that a strong majority of patients were interested in receiving written instruction sheets with their medication, especially information about the risks of medicines (Morris and Groft, 1982). Although patients expressed interest in large amounts of risk disclosure, FDA concluded that informational content of the PPI should be specified on a case by case basis. The important messages for each PPI should be tailored to address the specific problems patients faced using particular medication.

FDA developed and tested several prototype PPIs in a variety of research studies: small focus groups of eight to ten patients to obtain global reactions and open-ended remarks; pilot tests using college students to test how variations in format influenced knowledge and understanding of the material; and large scale studies of outpatients to examine attitudes, knowledge and clinical effects caused by PPI style variation. Several features of the PPIs were systematically varied in these studies to test questions about how to design an optimal PPI. For example:

PPI length: how long should the PPI be and what type of details should be added to the document?;

Readability level: should reading levels be kept at a specified grade level and, if so, how does one assure readability?;

Nature of risk disclosure: should specific and detailed risks be disclosed or should general warnings be added?;

Overall format, should the information be presented in the paragraph form or should an outline format be used?

The overall finding from these studies was that there are no simple rules for writing PPIs. Rather, there are trade-offs in PPI design. For example, if PPIs are designed to have a low reading level the informational content may be understandable but subjects viewed the document as uninteresting and felt it was written for children (Morris, Thilman and Myers, 1980). Short PPIs led to better recall of facts whereas long PPIs led to better integration of that material (Morris and Kanouse, 1980). Drafting PPIs required that each document had to be written with a specific audience in mind, to address a limited number of specific learning objectives (prioritizing information in the document, not deleting it) and tested to make sure that it achieved its intended communication goals.

In general, PPIs were found to produce neither the most hoped for goals of it benefactors nor the most feared effects predicted by its critics. Knowledge about the drug, especially less commonly known information such as side effects and risks, was improved for people obtaining written information. People liked receiving the information. However, behavioral effects were minimal. Except for short term (antibiotic) regimens, compliance was not improved by written instructions unless the written information was combined with additional social support and motivational interventions. On the other hand, people receiving PPIs were no more likely to refuse therapy, ask for refunds, or suffer the side effects listed in the brochure (Kanouse, Berry, Hayes-Roth, Rogers and Winkler, 1981).

Phase three - the "break-up"

Results of the evaluation studies provided fuel for both critics and advocates of PPIs. During the final weeks of the Carter Administration, FDA issued final regulations calling for a three year PPI pilot program covering ten drug classes. A broad sampling of drugs was covered and a full scale evaluation was planned to assure that sufficient data would be available for deciding whether or not to continue the program.

However, once the Reagan Administration took office, the PPI pilot program was immediately put on hold. Additional hearings were held in Washington, D. C., in front of the newly appointed FDA Commissioner, Dr. Arthur Hayes. Two major announcements were made at these hearings that dramatically influenced the PPI program. First, Ciba Geigy Pharmaceuticals proclaimed that the private sector could do a better job of patient education if unleashed from the threat of federal regulations and organized so that a concerted and coordinated effort could be undertaken. To provide the organizational impetus, Ciba Geigy pledged a million dollars to form the National Council of Patient Information and Education (NCPIE). This group was subsequently formed and still exists today with former congressman Paul Rogers as its director and over 200 public and private sector organizations constituting its membership.

Secondly, the American Medical Association (AMA) announced that it was undertaking its own initiative to provide patient education leaflets to physicians. The PMI (Patient Medication Instruction) program was later started with funding provided by the AMA and several pharmaceutical companies. An extensive mailing of sample leaflets was combined with public service advertisements directed to physicians and patients. Over 50 drug classes were covered in the initial phase and it grew to cover all of the major drug classes. Physicians could order supplies of PMIs for a minimal cost.

With these two major private sector initiatives, combined with many other patient education initiatives by other health professional associations and pharmaceutical companies, the FDA withdrew the PPI pilot program. FDA continued to provide research and consultative services to the private sector, primarily through NCPIE. Volunteerism, rather than regulation, was viewed as the primary method for providing patients with information about prescription drugs.

Phase four - the maturing relationship

As might be expected, consumer advocates who had favored PPI regulations became critics of FDA and private sector voluntary initiatives. However, even the strongest critics were impressed by the sheer number of voluntary programs introduced. It appeared that the private sector, now unencumbered by the threat of federal intervention, could indeed provide a wide variety of patient education materials. These materials could be better targeted to suit the needs of individual patients than a single required document that would have been mandated by federal regulations.

The pharmaceutical industry, which had long resisted drafting and distributing patient information on their products, began to distribute leaflets describing the medication to physicians as part of their promotional materials. Currently, it is the exception, rather than the rule, for a brand name product not to have a patient information brochure (Morris and Tyson, 1985).

However, evaluations of private sector initiatives have focused on the "production" side of the PPI equation. When FDA began to look on the "distribution" side, quite a different picture emerged. Although many different organizations were producing many different drug information leaflets, a relatively small percentage of patients seemed to be receiving any of these documents. A national survey undertaken in 1985 indicated that although 25% of patients reported receiving some written information at the pharmacy when they picked up their medication, this information was usually in the form of small stickers affixed to the medication vial. Only 6% reported receiving a brochure and 7% an instruction sheet. Only 9% reported receiving written information at the physician's office (Morris, Grossman, Barkdoll and Gordon, 1986). These percentages were almost identical to data collected in 1982, with the only noticeable increase in the 1985 data being an increase in the provision of sticker labels at the pharmacy (Morris, Grossman, Barkdoll, Gordon and Soviero, 1983).

A more precise measure of pharmacy distribution of PPIs under voluntary conditions was provided by an evaluation of the patient education program initiated for propoxyphene by Eli Lilly, makers of Darvon. Following the accumulation of evidence that overdose of propoxyphene in combination with other psychoactive substances could cause fatal consequences, a multifaceted patient education program was initiated which included the distribution of a PPI to pharmacies. Although a telephone survey of pharmacists indicated that 90% said they received the shipment of PPIs and 85% said they had it in stock, when observers posing as patients had prescriptions filled, only 5% received the leaflet spontaneously, and 32% received one if requested (Morris and Groft, 1982). As seen above, the comparable figures for mandated PPIs for conjugated estrogens were 39% spontaneous delivery, 89% if requested.

Whereas, the distribution rate for mandatory PPIs was low, the rate for voluntary ones appeared paltry. Neither method seemed to provide assurance that a consumer would receive a necessary warning message. Thus, FDA moved away from regulations as a means of warning delivery and turned toward packaging solutions to assure that PPIs were delivered. Recent efforts in the regulation of Accutane, indicated for cystic acne, and Cytotec, indicated for protection against ulcers caused by non-steroidal antiinflammatory drugs (e.g., aspirin), demonstrate FDA's current thinking about PPIs.

Although Accutane is a uniquely effective drug it is also a known teratogen. When first approved in the United States, a patient brochure was drafted that explicitly warned users that birth defects were likely if the drug was used during pregnancy. Copies of the brochure were distributed by the manufacturer and pharmacists were requested to distribute them to patients obtaining a prescription. After several years of marketing, a review of epidemiological evidence indicated that a surprisingly large number of children with birth defects were born to women who had taken Accutane.

Although FDA considered removing the drug from the market, it was decided that the benefit to risk ratio for people who were not pregnant was positive and that the drug should remain on the market. However, several steps were taken to assure that women who have the potential to become pregnant were fully informed about the absolute contraindication of using Accutane during pregnancy or becoming pregnant while taking Accutane.

Rather than relying on a voluntary patient brochure, a PPI was required as part of the patient labeling. As this labeling was required for a single product, rather than a class of products, the labeling could be instituted without the issuance of regulations (a time consuming process that requires the issuance of a proposal, public debate, and a final regulation). The distribution system for the medication was changed as Accutane became prepackaged in unit-of-use blister packs. The new package has extra cardboard panels which contain an extensive warning message and symbols to indicate the pregnancy warning.

Furthermore, the PPI was designed as only one aspect of a pregnancy prevention program. Physicians are supplied with brochures, checklists, referral telephone numbers, educational materials, and a patient information/consent sheet to help assure that female patients are fully informed about the risks of using the drug.

It is hoped that this combination of interventions will help reduce Accutane pregnancies.

Cytotec is also a drug that has a fairly unique indication; however, it too has predictable, severe side effects. Cytotec is known to cause spontaneous abortions and must not be used by women who are pregnant or may become pregnant. Like Accutane, patient labeling was required for Cytotec. A small leaflet (in English and Spanish) warning women not to take the drug if pregnant is attached to unit-of-use bottles. In addition, there is a "do not use if pregnant" warning on the bottle top and on the outer package. There is also a warning symbol (a silhouette with a pregnant woman with a red line across it) placed on the bottle.

FDA currently views the need for PPIs on a case by case basis. On rare occasions, where special warnings are needed, PPIs are required. When broad scale implementation of PPIs was first contemplated in the mid 1970's, the (1) development and (2) distribution of patient information sheets was seen as presenting two major problems. Today, numerous examples of informative patient information materials exist. The public has become more sophisticated and desirous of patient information. However, effective distribution systems, other than costly packing solutions, remain a severe constraint. In foreign countries, where drugs are prepackaged in unit-of-use containers, inclusion of PPIs are not perceived as presenting major logistical barriers.

Assessment of PPI Effects

PPIs have been touted as remarkable successes and as serious failures; as facilitory and as disruptive; as efficient and as costly. All of these conclusions are, of course, correct. Any assessment of the PPI depends ultimately on the observer's expectations and point of view. Furthermore, with an intervention as flexible as a PPI (in terms of content, distribution method, and the environment in which it is received), that may be differentially conceived as addressing a wide range of purposes, and implemented in a well or ill conceived manner, overly general conclusions can be inherently misleading.

Therefore, any assessment of the PPI must have appropriate caveats about limits to its conclusions and the necessary and sufficient conditions leading to observed effects.

There are two major classes of effects that are usually considered when evaluating PPIs. First are the communications effects. Many of the studies assessing PPIs have included a knowledge test to measure, what, if anything, patients learn from PPIs. Other questions such as "are PPIs read?", "can the information in a PPI be understood?", and "does the PPI meaningfully influence attitudes and decisions about proper drug use?" are addressed less often by objective evaluation but are, nevertheless, important to frame the basis for a full evaluation of the PPI as a communications vehicle.

The second class of questions are those assessing behavioral outcomes. Assessment of the PPI's influence on regimen adherence is the most frequent focus of behavioral evaluation studies. However, other effects, such as influences on the doctor-patient relationship, and assessment of unintended effects, such as the occurrence of returned prescriptions and suggestion induced side effects, have been studied in a small number of formal evaluations. Since we have already reviewed some of this literature, we will highlight evaluation research on certain areas not already covered.

Patient knowledge

Ley and Morris (1984) reviewed 32 studies that examined the effect of written information on patient knowledge and found only one study where there was no knowledge gain comparing subjects receiving a PPI to those that did not receive one. Although the weight of evidence clearly supports the PPI as an educational vehicle, many of the studies examined in the Ley and Morris review suffered from two methodological problems.

First, in the majority of studies the PPI was not the only educational intervention. The counseling of a health professional, the use of special packaging, reminder stickers, or audiovisual aids were also used in many of these studies in an effort to improve patients' knowledge about their medication and their condition. Therefore, educational gains may not be attributable solely to the PPI. Fortunately, there are a few studies that examined the PPI without additional educational interventions. In a more in depth review, Morris and Halperin (1979) found that in seven of eight studies that did not include additional interventions, knowledge was improved. However, it appeared that knowledge improvement was not always obtained on all measurement scales. Rather, improvement tended to occur on scales that measured knowledge about drug effects, such as precautions and side effects, that are not routinely covered in verbal counseling or were known by most patients.

The second consideration when evaluating this literature relates to generalizing results. It is not surprising that providing a PPI to patients as part of a study leads to improved knowledge scores. Frequently these studies took place in a clinic where the health professional provided directions to read the document and patients knew that they would be called on at some time later to answer questions about the document.

Does knowledge reliably increase under more natural conditions? Two broad scale evaluations provide some suggestive evidence that knowledge may be improved with PPIs in more naturalistic environments. First, in the FDA survey of oral conceptive users 54% of the women currently taking the pill could identify the danger of blood clots as the most serious side effect of using the pill (Morris, Mazis and Gordon, 1977). The respondents were recruited via a household canvass and were not pre-informed about the interview. The 54% knowledge rate seems relatively high compared to other studies of the general level of side effect communication from health professionals to patients. Unfortunately, there was no control group in this study and we do not know if knowledge is attributable to the PPI or some other cause.

Second, in a study conducted by the Rand Corporation under an FDA contract, 69 community pharmacies in the Los Angeles area were recruited to distribute specially designed PPIs for three drugs: an antibiotic (erythromycin), a sleeping pill (Dalmane), and conjugated estrogens (Kanouse, Berry, Hayes-Roth, Rogers and Winkler, 1981). Although still an experimental design, the breadth of distribution sites and "real world" features of the study provide a more generalizable set of data. The authors concluded that PPIs led to reliable gains in drug knowledge. For two of the drugs, erythromycin and Dalmane, there were no-PPI control groups. Erythromycin patients who received a PPI were better able to answer questions about how the drug worked and Dalmane subjects who received a PPI were more aware of the dangers of drug interactions and pregnancy contraindications compared to patients prescribed the medication who did not receive a PPI.

Regimen adherence

Studies assessing PPIs' effects on improving patient compliance with prescription drug regimens have shown mixed results. In the Ley and Morris (1984) review, 15 of 25 studies showed improvement in compliance rates; however, as in the case of the knowledge results, many of these studies had multiple interventions. Examining the same data base, Morris and Halperin (1979) concluded that PPIs may be effective for antibiotics where a simple message (i.e., "finish all your medication") requests a short term (i.e., ten day) behavior change. However, for medication that requires long term maintenance, the PPI in and of itself has not been shown to be effective at improving compliance. Kanouse, Berry, Hayes-Roth, Rogers and Winkler (1981) found no improvements in compliance for any of the drugs they studied, including erythromycin.

Reviews of patient compliance interventions have not revealed any low cost intervention that reliably improves medication taking behavior (Haynes, 1985). However, all of the studies that have examined compliance interventions have utilized a clinical trials approach, enrolling several hundred patients at most in any test. One may speculate that in order to improve compliance with medication regimens, not only are informational interventions needed, but so are motivational interventions and skill training (Mazzuca, 1982). If effective at all, a PPI is likely to have informational effects and be relatively ineffective at supplying the necessary motivational elements, or providing the feedback necessary for skill training. One may speculate further that a PPI, or any other low cost compliance promoting strategy (i.e., a strategy that does not require the continued personal involvement of a health professional), will be effective only for a small number of patients. PPIs will lead to behavior change only for patients who require only information to change long term behavior (no additional skill training or motivational impetus is needed). Large scale population based studies may be necessary to find a sufficient number of these individuals. Unfortunately, reliable measures of compliance are not easily applied to population based studies and this speculation may be difficult to verify or refute. Furthermore, even if true, this line of reasoning assumes that the PPI is a weak intervention at best and cannot be assumed to be an effective long term compliance promoting strategy.

Doctor-patient relationship

PPIs have been criticized because they would: (1) decrease the number and length of doctor visits (thereby interfering with the doctor-patient relationship) or (2) increase the number and length of doctor visits (thereby increasing health care costs). From the existing studies, neither of these effects occur to a great extent. In both the oral contraceptive and Rand studies, there was no significant change reported in the number or length of doctor visits. However, both studies indicated that the content of the interaction was influenced by the PPI. Patients reported a greater likelihood that the drug was discussed during the doctor visit. It is not clear if this conversation was cued by the patient's questions or if the doctor anticipated problems with patients who received the PPI and sought to head off difficulties that the patient might have understanding or interpreting the PPI.

Returned prescriptions

One concern is that patients would read the PPI, become frightened, and refuse to take their medication. Some have speculated that this might lead to an increase in the number of prescriptions returned for a refund. Although several estimates of the number of prescription returns have been made, the only data bearing on this issue comes from the Rand study which found only three of 2,000 prescriptions that were issued with a PPI were returned for a refund. There are no data on baseline rates of prescription returns so evaluation of the cost increase, if any, cannot be made. Furthermore, it is unclear if a returned prescription is a positive or a negative health outcome. It is entirely possible that patients who return prescriptions are making rational decisions on the basis of information in the PPI and consultation with their doctor. Any assessment of returned prescriptions should ascertain if the prescription is returned because of an irrational fear or valid information.

Conclusion

Thus, PPIs may be useful to communicate some elements of treatment, especially the risks of treatment. As physicians may be uncomfortable or unwilling to disclose serious but rare unavoidable risks, the PPI may be a useful tool. PPIs have been used primarily as a vehicle of risk communication. They do not appear to be as effective causing behavioral changes, either positive ones (such as improving regimen adherence) or negative ones (frightening patients into refusing their treatment). The effects of the PPI on the doctor-patient relationship are an important element to consider. The oral contraceptive study suggests that the length of time devoted to drug discussions may rise. Some doctors, anticipating the distribution of PPIs, may adjust their script to provide a fuller context for the patient to evaluate the risks and benefits of treatment. In this case, the PPI may be viewed by the patient as supporting the therapeutic relationship. It is possible that other doctors may fail to mention the PPI or wish not to disclose risks. For these doctors, the PPI may be a disruptive influence. Thus, the PPI may be viewed as a limited tool in risk communication that may aid or hinder therapeutic relationships depending on how it is used.

Direct Advertising of Prescription Drugs

Traditionally, the promotion of prescription drugs has been limited to the health professionals who prescribe and dispense them. However, in recent years, several pharmaceutical companies have expressed an interest in promoting prescription medication directly to the public.

Manufacturer rationale

There are several reasons for manufacturers to communicate directly with the public. For example, unless consumers know that a new product exists, they may refrain from visiting the doctor. Merrill-Dow, makers of Seldane (a nonsedating antihistamine), found it beneficial to advertise that the doctor can prescribe nonsedating hay fever medication. Secondly, direct promotion to the consumer may speed the adoption of a new product, especially if the condition is underdiagnosed. Hoechst-Roussel, makers of Trental (a drug that makes blood flow more easily), created commercials that inform elderly consumers that pain in the leg while walking may be due to "intermittent claudication," the medical indication for their drug. If individuals recognize a medical condition they may view it as treatable and be more likely to visit their doctor. Thirdly, if a product has a price advantage, the consumer may be more likely to request it at the pharmacy. Lexis, makers of a birth control pill, ran advertisements informing consumers that their product was identical to other oral contraceptives but sold at a cheaper price.

Risk disclosure requirements

A major problem for drug manufacturers desiring to promote prescription drugs directly to consumers is FDA regulations regarding promotion. Unlike other consumer products, the promotion of prescription medication must comply with the requirements of the Food, Drug, and Cosmetic Act. To be in compliance with this law, advertisements must meet two standards. First, the advertisements must not be false or misleading. FDA interprets the false and misleading standard quite broadly. An advertisement may be considered false and misleading if it does not reveal facts that may be material to the prescribing decision. Furthermore, advertisements must be "fairly balanced"; risk information or product limitations must be disclosed so that the prescriber of the product understands important limitations to the claims being made.

Secondly, advertisements for prescription medication must contain a "brief summary" of contraindications, warnings, and precautions. The "brief summary" requirement is met by most firms by reprinting or distributing the major sections of the product labeling. This disclosure frequently entails a full page of small print in a medical journal. In audiovisual advertisements, this disclosure is made either by distributing product labeling information at the time of the broadcast or running a "crawl" of this information following the broadcast (usually in the early morning hours) and assuring that viewers of the broadcast have access to the prescribing information (by distributing a book of prescribing information to all doctors and having a toll free number where consumers may obtain the information).

Given these broad scale disclosure requirements, prescription drug manufacturers have, for the most part, decided to skirt the FDA requirements by promoting their products indirectly. Rather than create advertisements that mention and promote the drug, these advertisements do not mention the names of the product, or prescription drugs per se. For the most part, these are viewed as advertisements that promote help seeking for particular conditions. In all cases, there are therapies other than prescription medication that could be utilized. They qualify as help seeking rather than prescription drug advertisements. Thus, these advertisements are outside the FDA's regulatory purview. The one exception is advertisements that promote price, where risk disclosures are not required as long as no health claims are made about the product.

There have been a few examples where companies have run a prescription drug advertisement that contained the disclosures required by FDA. In all these instances, the promotion has occurred in print where the brief summaries were reprinted next to the advertisement. The prescribing information reprinted has been based on physician labeling. Thus, the risk information disclosed to the consumer was long, complex, and perhaps unintelligible to most lay persons. Recently, Lakeside Pharmaceuticals developed a consumer oriented print advertisement for Nicorette, an antismoking treatment, that contained prescribing information that was based on physician information translated into lay language. Also, Upjohn, makers of Rogaine, a baldness remedy, ran newspaper advertisements with translated prescribing information.

Only a few companies have run print advertisements that qualify as prescription drug advertisements directed to consumers. There have been several television commercials developed to promote products directly to consumers; however, none qualify as prescription drug advertisements. (The one exception, a television advertisement for Rufen, an antiinflammatory drug, was run only once on a test basis and FDA objected to the commercial.) The risk disclosure requirements present a formidable barrier for manufacturers wishing to direct television advertisements directly to consumers.

Political environment

As might be expected a number of groups have suggested that FDA modify its regulations to make direct advertisements to consumers more easily attainable. Also, as might be expected, there has be counter-debate by opponents of direct-to-consumer advertising suggesting that the de facto barrier of FDA regulations remain in place to discourage direct advertising. The proponents of direct advertising suggest that more advertising could increase the consumers' role in health care, improve dialogue with the doctor, increase compliance with medication regimens, decrease costs of pharmaceuticals through increased demand, and generally serve consumers' right to know about the drugs they take. Opponents suggest that the exact opposite would happen. It would interfere with the doctor-patient relationship, promotion would confuse the consumer, lead to the misuse of medications, increase drug prices, and prompt consumers to "trivialize" the advertised medication (failing to recognize important risks and limitations about the product).

In recent years two major "players" have entered the DTCA debate. At the urging of the major television networks, a consortium of advertising agencies, communications organizations, pharmaceutical companies has been formed to promote direct to consumer advertising. Secondly, three influential Congressmen: Dingle, Waxman, and Marke, have written letters to the networks urging them not to lobby for direct to consumer advertising. In response to this congressional pressure, the consortium has refocused its efforts to study the impact of direct to consumer advertising.

Survey data

The need for study is, of course, essential to assure that public policy be developed in an enlightened fashion. Although there has been much debate about DTCA there has been surprisingly little scientific scrutiny. Several surveys have obtained health professional and consumer attitudes about direct advertising (Columbia Broadcasting System, 1984; American Druggist, 1982; Ruder, Finn, and Rotman, 1985). Generally, health professionals have strong reservations about the concept but appear to be accepting when shown particular advertisements. Consumers vary in their response depending on how the question is asked.

Attitudes about DTCA are not well formed because people have no clear idea about what constitutes the "stimulus object" under evaluation. Without clear exemplars or prototypes, people can only imagine what is meant by consumer advertising. When shown examples, individuals tend to rely on these examples to form their opinion. Without examples, the way in which the question is phrased dictates measured attitudes. For example, in a survey by Rudder, Finn, and Rotman (1985), people were asked "if more information through consumer advertising were available about prescription drugs, do you think you would be better informed about the drugs you take or do you feel that advertising would not make a difference?" Half (50%) of the respondents said they would be better informed. By focusing on the "more information" delivered through advertising and asking only if people would be better informed, the question emphasized only the positive elements of advertising and failed to solicit any negative views. Similarly, questions that focus on advertising without acknowledging positive contributions would be likely to solicit negative biases. Thus, without clear examples and unbiased surveys, polls soliciting people's views must be questioned about their validity.

Sales experience

Perhaps more important than polling data are studies that measure consumer response to direct advertising. The most direct measures come from experience with consumer directed advertising.

Gross sales increases have been shown for some of the products promoted with health care seeking commercials (e.g., Nicorette, Seldane) whereas other products have not been as successfully promoted (e.g., Tagamet (an ulcer drug), and Rogaine (for hair loss)). In an evaluation of a test consumer advertising campaign for Rufen run in Florida, 34% of a sample of arthritis suffers said they were aware of Rufen and half (53%) of the aware group said they first became aware through television advertising. Thus, television promotion appears able to promote brand awareness whether it results in behavioral actions (visiting the doctor, obtaining the medication, etc.) is more problematic.

Risk Disclosure in Television and Magazines

While brand name awareness and sales are the important issues for manufacturers of prescription drugs, an important public policy question is whether the FDA risk disclosure requirements can or should be applied to consumer advertising. The risk disclosure requirements presently applied are based on a law directed to physicians who make prescribing decisions. A busy physician may be unable to locate prescribing information and may appreciate the easily availability of risk information disclosed within prescription drug advertisements. Since the consumer does not make prescribing decisions, what role would, or should, risk information play in the prescribing process?

Purpose of risk disclosure

Both proponents and opponents of DTCA suggest that the doctor-patient relationship is paramount to medication prescribing. Direct to consumer promotion should improve, rather than interrupt, the prescribing process. Thus, risk information, if it has any role, should improve the dialogue between doctor and patient. Improvement in this case may be regarded as focusing the dialogue on treatment, leading to more question-asking about the medication on behalf of the patient, and perhaps result in more appropriate prescribing for patients.

However, these goals lead to two differing opinions about the form of risk disclosure in advertisements. Some suggest that a generally phrased risk disclosure (e.g., "ask your doctor about the side effects of this drug") would serve as an adequate method of providing risk information to consumers. Others suggest that a more stringent standard be applied, incorporating specific risk disclosure information into the advertisement (e.g., "this drug causes gout").

FDA study

To test the effects of risk disclosure variations on consumers' knowledge and behavior, FDA conducted a test of prototype prescription drug advertisements directed to consumers (Morris and Millstein, 1984). Both television and magazine advertisements were created for two fictitious drugs: "Diroven," an antihypertensive drug that was worn as a skin patch, and "Artomine," an antiarthritic drug taken once-a-day.

The method of disclosing risks was varied in these advertisements. First, the length of risk disclosure was varied so that some of the advertisements contained two risk statements and some contained four risk statements. Secondly, the specificity of risk disclosure was manipulated so that some of the advertisements contained general, "see your doctor" risk disclosures and others contained more specific risk statements. Thirdly, the degree to which risk information was emphasized within the advertisements was varied. For some of the advertisements the risk information was integrated within the advertisement in a routine fashion while for other advertisements, the risk information was made to stand out from the background using audio or visual cues to make the risk information discernable.

Individuals were recruited in four cities using random digit dialing techniques. Subjects were asked to come to a central facility to view some health information materials. After subjects arrived at the facility, they either viewed a videotape with the test commercials embedded or read a magazine with the test advertisements reprinted. In addition to varying the length, specificity, and emphasis of risk disclosure in an orthogonal fashion, control advertisements were created that contained either no risk information or disclosed an extreme amount of risk information by attaching a video scroll or brief summary disclosure (i.e., the boiler plate risk disclosure that exists in physician advertising). Subjects were next asked to fill out a questionnaire that measured knowledge and attitudes related to the advertisement. They were debriefed and paid $20.00 for participating in the study.

Knowledge results

The major dependent knowledge measures taken were the nature and extent of risk information recalled, relative to the recall of benefit information. Comparing the television and magazine conditions presents many uncontrollable conditions. Although there was better recall in the television condition, this is clearly attributable to viewing conditions. When subjects viewing the magazines were informed to pay particular attention to the advertisements, information from the advertisement was recalled much more fully. Interestingly, there was a higher level of recall of incorrect information in the magazine advertisement than in the forced exposure television commercial (Morris, Brinberg, Klinberg, Rivera and Millstein, 1986). Again, this is attributable to the forced exposure in the television conditions compared to a magazine readership situation that permitted skimming of the advertising material.

In terms of the television advertisement, subjects who viewed advertisements with longer and more specific risk disclosures had better recall of risk information. The method of risk emphasis led to differing recall of risk information. When risk information was presented in a dual modality (in both the audio and video portions using superimposed graphics with the warning messages appearing on screen when the announcer read them), there was an increased recall of risk information. However, when the risk information was grouped together to make it more distinctive, there was a reduced recall of risk information (perhaps due to stimulus overload conditions).

There were few effects of risk disclosure format on the recall of benefit information. However, in the risk specificity conditions, there was some indication that the presentation of vivid risks detracted from the communication of product benefits. Viscusi and

Magat (1987) found similar trade-offs in the processing of warning messages in product labels for prototype chemical warning labels. The internal primes of a vivid warning message may indeed direct attention to one aspect of a message and away from other elements of the message.

In terms of comprehension of risk and benefit information, there was a direct relationship between the communication of risk information and resultant knowledge (as measured by a true-false test). Advertisements that contained specific risks led to greater comprehension of that risk information. However, advertisements that contained general risk information did not improve comprehension of the general risk information. It appeared that the general risk information was already well known to subjects.

Attitude results

The attitude data suggest that subjects viewing the general risk advertisements had a more favorable evaluation of the drug and the advertisement. Thus, the advertisements containing general risk information were more likely to be perceived as reassuring rather than conveying risk information (Morris, Brinberg, Klinberg, Millstein and Rivera, 1986). In a conceptual replication of this study using audience testing arrangement, 3,374 individuals recruited to view television programming were shown one of the television test advertisements and provide emotional reactions to the advertisement via a semantic differential. Specific and longer advertisements were perceived as more irritating than the shorter and the general risk advertisements (Morris, Ruffner and Klinberg, 1985).

Conclusion

These studies suggest that specific disclosures are more informative about the risks of the product. However, they may also distract from the communication of product benefits and consumers do not particularly like advertisements containing specific risks. General risk information, on the other hand, is perceived as reassuring more than informative. Given the purpose of the legal requirements for risk disclosure, it is unclear how general risk information could serve either the "balancing" or "disclosure" purposes specified for risk disclosures.

It is not known if general or specific risk disclosures would lead to more focused physician-patient interactions and better prescribing. Clearly, more research is needed to understand behavioral practices engendered by different risk disclosures. Recently, the DTCA Consortium has proposed "market testing" of prescription drug advertisements that would examine the influence of the advertisements on physician-patient encounters and on other elements as well. Real world testing of such advertisements would aid in understanding the impact, if any, of such advertisements on patients and their providers.

Implications

Patient package inserts and direct advertising of prescription drugs to consumers have been two extremely controversial topics. Evidently, warning information disclosure raises political, economic, and ethical apprehension for those concerned with health care communications.

The PPI debate has waned as FDA has adopted a practice of issuing PPIs only in rare instances when the product's marketing necessitates extraordinary warning disclosure conditions. The use of a PPI as a warning label, rather than as a general education document to disclose risks about all drugs, has had both beneficial and negative ramifications. On the positive side, the PPI can "signal" consumers that special attention is necessary when using these special drugs. The consumer is unlikely to become habituated to prescription drug warnings. On the other hand, the consumer has not become routinely educated about the risks of using prescription drugs. There has been little societal impact of increased, routine risk disclosure that may have provided a better basis for patients understanding the risk-benefit trade-offs incumbent when using prescription medication. Tracking general risks perception in Europe (compared to the United States) may help evaluate whether the routine distribution of PPIs influences these perceptions, tolerance for risk, and search activity (question-asking of physicians).

Direct advertising to consumers has raised a different set of concerns. Interestingly, the same arguments offered in support, or against, PPIs have been offered in regards to DTCA---but by the opposite set of critics. Unlike PPIs, however, there is very little data to help discern the influence of this potentially profound influence on patient and consumer perceptions, knowledge, and behavior.

Many critics would like to ban DTCA. Under current conditions there is a de facto ban as most advertisements are viewed as "help seeking" advertisements that do not name or promote specific prescription medication. This has left a void for the marketing manager that wishes to use a "pull through" distribution strategy, getting patients to request the name of their drug.

Given the limits on advertising, several firms have turned to using public relations to get the name of the product in front of the consumer. Recently, Ciba Geigy hired former baseball player Mickey Mantle to promote a new antiarthritic medication (Deutsch, 1989). The ultimate outlet for public relations messages is the general content of media rather than paid for and identified space or time that serves as the outlet for advertising. General content of media is not processed with the same degree of skepticism as advertising. People are less sensitive to source effects in general media content and are more likely to accept and integrate these message into their schema compared to advertising messages (Morris, Brinberg and Plimpton, 1984).

The degree to which marketers are willing to incorporate risk information into television commercials is open to conjecture. Clearly, they would prefer general warning messages. On the other hand, the degree to which regulatory agencies will accept vague risk disclosures is also an open question.

Endnote

Life is full of risks and dwelling on what can go wrong serves little rational purpose. Yet, we all need to cope with the threats we face. As patients we are dependent on, and vulnerable to, the therapies we receive. Whether we actively approach or passively deny the risks of therapy, we need to have the opportunity to understand, master, and control our fate. Ethical arguments, reinforced by court rulings, do not provide health professionals the option to withhold important warnings, except in extreme cases. Risk communication serves both the patient and the doctor in the long run.

The problem faced by risk communicators is how to convey important risks in a helpful fashion. Our view is that risk communication is a long term process. Providing opportunities and cues to discuss risks in a supportive environment is the best strategy. It is unrealistic to ask doctors to disclose any but the most important risks. Doctors are willing to disclose preventable risks but rare, unavoidable risks are frequently uncommunicated unless forced through an informed consent procedure.

Providing patients with print or audiovisual materials that describe risks and spur questions may increase risk communication. Effective distribution strategies for such materials await innovation and commitment. Only time will tell if patient demand and marketplace forces will increase risk information flow to consumers.

References

Aaronson, L., Mural, C. & Pfoutz, S.: Seeking information: Where do pregnant women go? Health Education Quarterly, 1988, 15, 335-345.

Abram, M.: Making Health Care Decisions: The Ethical and Legal Implications of Informed Consent in the Patient-Practitioner Relationship. The President's Commission for the Study of Ethical Problems in Medicine and Biomedical and Behavioral Research. Government Printing Office: Washington, D.C., 1982.

Alba, J. & Hutchinson, J.: Dimensions of consumer expertise. Journal of Consumer Research, 1987, 13, 411-454.

American Druggist: Two-thirds of RPh's and MD's object to makers' promotion of Rx drugs to the public. American Druggist, 1982, 186, 14-21.

Amir, M.: Considerations guiding physicians when informing cancer patients. Social Science and Medicine, 1987, 24, 741-748.

Anderson, J., Dodman, S., Kopelman, M., & Fleming, A.: Patient information recall in a rheumatology clinic. Rheumatology and Rehabilitation, 1979, 17, 18-22.

Anderson, L., DeVellis, B. & DeVellis, R.: Effects of modeling on patient communication, satisfaction, and knowledge. Medical Care, 1987, 25, 1044-1056.

Arkes, H. & Harkness, A.: Effect of making a diagnosis on subsequent recognition of symptoms. Journal of Experimental Psychology: Human Learning and Memory, 1980, 6, 568-575.

Ashworth, C., Williamson, P. & Montano, D.: A scale to measure physician beliefs about psychosocial aspects of patient care. Social Science and Medicine, 1984, 19, 1235-1238.

Avery, J.: How the medical "lawsuit pie" is cut: Lawyers tell what turns some patients litigious. Medical Malpractice Prevention, 1986, 1, 35-37.

Bain, D.: The content of physician-patient communication in family practice. The Journal of Family Practice, 1979, 8, 745-753.

Baker, M.: Americans and their doctors. New York: Louis Harris and Associates, 1985.

Barofsky, I.: Compliance, adherence and the therapeutic alliance - steps in the development of self care. Social Science and Medicine, 1978, 12, 369-376.

Beatty, S. & Smith, S.: External search effort: An investigation across several product categories. Journal of Consumer Research, 1987, 14, 83-95.

Bechtel, G. & Ribera, J.: Risk acceptability in segments with distinct value orientations. Advances in Consumer Research, 1983, 10, 590-595.

Becker, M. & Maiman, L.: Sociobehavioral determinants of compliance with health and medical care recommendations. Medical Care, 1975, 13, 10-24.

Beeson, D. & Golbus, M.: Decision making: Whether or not to have prenatal diagnosis and abortion for X-linked conditions. American Journal of Medical Genetics, 1985, 20, 107-114.

Berwick, D. & Weinstein, M.: What do patients value? Willingness to pay for ultrasound in normal pregnancy. Medical Care, 1985, 23, 881-893.

Bishop, G.: Illness cognition in response to AIDS. Talk given at the American Psychological Association Meeting, Atlanta, Ga., August, 1988.

Boreham, P. & Gibson, D.: The information process in private medical consultations: A preliminary investigation. Social Science and Medicine, 1978, 12, 409-416.

Borgida, E. & Nisbett, R.: The differential impact of abstract vs. concrete information on decisions. Journal of Applied Social Psychology, 1977, 7, 258-271.

Bower, G., Black, J. & Turner, T.: Scripts in memory for text. Cognitive Psychology, 1979, 11, 177-220.

Bower, G. & Clark-Meyers, G.: Memory for scripts with organized vs. randomized presentations. British Journal of Psychology, 1980, 71, 369-377.

Boyle, C.: Difference between patients' and doctors' interpretation of some common medical terms. British Journal of Medicine, 1970, 2, 286-289.

Boyle, J.: Patient information and prescription drugs: Parallel surveys of physicians and pharmacists. New York: Louis Harris and Associates, 1983.

Bransford, J. & Johnson, M.: Contextual prerequisites for understanding: Some investigations of comprehension and recall. Journal of Verbal Learning and Verbal Behavior, 1972, 11, 717-726.

Brody, D.: An analysis of patient recall of their therapeutic regimens. Journal of Chronic Diseases, 1980, 33, 57-63.

Brown, S.: Spotting the patients most likely to sue. Medical Economics, 1983, 66, 98-101.

Brown, S. & Swartz, T.: Consumer medial complaint behavior: Determinants of and alternatives to malpractice litigation. Journal of Public Policy and Marketing. 1984, 3, 85-98.

Brushwood, D. & Simonsmeier, L.: Drug information for patients: Duties of the manufacturer, pharmacist, physician, and hospital. The Journal of Legal Medicine, 1986, 7, 279-340.

Bryant, G. & Norman, G.: Expressions of probability - words and numbers. New England Journal of Medicine. 1980, 302, 411.

Buchsbaum, D.: Reassurance reconsidered. Social Science and Medicine, 1986, 23, 423-427.

Bullman, W. & Rowland, F.: Directory of Prescription Drug Information and Education Programs and Resources. Washington, D.C.: National Council on Patient Information and Education, 1986.

Cantor, N., Mischel, W. & Schwartz, J.: A prototype analysis of psychological situations. Cognitive Psychology, 1982, 14, 45-77.

Carey, K. & Dogan, W.: Exploration of factors influencing physicians to refer patients for mental health services. Medical Care, 1971, 9, 55-66.

Carter, W., Inui, T., Kukull, W. & Haigh, V.: Outcome based doctor-patient interaction analysis. II Identifying effective provider and patient behavior. Medical Care, 1982, 20, 550-573.

Carver, C., Scheier, M. & Weintraub, J.: Assessing coping strategies: A theoretically based approach. Journal of Personality and Social Psychology, 1989, 56, 267-283.

Cartwright, A., Lucas, S. & O'Brien, M.: Some methodological problems in studying consultations in general practice. Journal of the Royal College of General Practitioners, 1976, 26, 894-906.

Cartwright, A. & Smith, C: Elderly People, Their Medicines, and Their Doctors. Routledge: London, 1988.

Cassileth, B., Zupkis, R., Sutton-Smith, K. & March, V.: Informed consent - why are its goals imperfectly realized? New England Journal of Medicine, 1980, 302, 896-900.

Christensen-Szalanski, J., Beck, D., Christensen-Szalanski, C. & Koepsell, T.: Effects of expertise and experience on risk judgments. Journal of Applied Psychology, 1983, 68, 278-284.

Christensen-Szalanski, J., Boyce, W., Harrell, H. & Gardner, M.: Circumcision and informed consent: Is more information always better? Medical Care, 1987, 25, 856-867.

Christensen-Szalanski, J. & Northcraft, G.: Patient compliance behavior: The effects of time on patients' values of treatment regimens. Social Science and Medicine, 1985, 21, 263-273.

Clarke, A. & Johnston, M.: Use of a medical "schema" in facilitating access to understanding in psychology. Medical Education, 1986, 20, 410-416.

Cohn, J. & Basu, K.: Alternative models of categorization: Toward a contingent processing framework. Journal of Consumer Research, 1987, 13, 455-471.

Columbia Broadcasting System: Prescription Drug Advertising: Issues & Perspectives. Columbia Broadcasting System: New York, 1984.

Conrad, P.: The meaning of medications: Another look at compliance. Social Science and Medicine. 1985, 20, 29-37.

Covello, V.: The perception of technological risks: A literature review. Technological Forecasting and Social Change, 1983, 23, 285-297.

Dance, K & Neufeld, R.: Aptitude-treatment interaction research in the clinical setting: A review of attempts to dispel the "patient uniformity" myth. Psychological Bulletin, 1988, 104, 192-213.

Danzon, P.: The frequency and severity of medical malpractice claims: new evidence. Law and Contemporary Problems, 1986, 49, 57-66.

Davis, M.: Physiologic, psychologic and demographic factors in patient compliance with doctors' orders. Medical Care, 1968, 6, 115-143.

Davitz, J.: My patients told me I was rude. Medical Economics, 1986, 69, 102-107.

Deutsch, C.: The brouhaha over drug ads. New York Times. 1989, 176, 7-10.

Diamond, G., Rozanski, A. & Steuer, M.: Playing doctor: Application of game theory to medical decision making. Journal of Chronic Disease, 1986, 39, 669-677.

Dodd, M.: Self-care for side effects in cancer chemotherapy: An assessment of nursing interventions - Part II. Cancer Nursing, 1983, 3, 63-67.

Dodd, M.: Measuring informational intervention for chemotherapy knowledge and self-care behavior. Research in Nursing and Health, 1984, 7, 43-50.

Eisenberg, J.: Sociologic influences on decision-making by clinicians. Annals of Internal Medicine, 1979, 90, 957-964.

Eisenberg, J., Kitz, D. & Webber, R.: Development and attitudes about sharing decision-making: A comparison of medical and surgical residents. Journal of Health and Social Behavior, 1983, 24, 85-90.

Engle, J., Blackwell, R. & Miniard, P.: Consumer Behavior. New York: Holt, Reinhart & Winston, 1986.

Epstein, S. & Clark, S.: Heart rate and skin conductance during experimentally induced anxiety - effects of anticipated noxious stimulation and experience. Journal of Experimental Psychology, 1970, 84, 105-112.

Eraker, S., Kirsch, J. & Becker, M.: Understanding and improving patient compliance. Annals of Internal Medicine, 1984, 100, 258-268.

Eraker, S. & Polister, P.: How decisions are reached: Physician and patient. Annals of Internal Medicine, 1982, 97, 262-268.

Eraker, S. & Sox, H.: An assessment of patient preferences for therapeutic outcomes. Medical Decision Making, 1981, 1, 29-39.

Eyesenck, M.: Anxiety, learning and memory: A reconceptualization. Journal of Research in Personality, 1979, 13, 362-385.

Faden, R., Becker, C., Lewis, C., Freeman, J. & Faden, A.: Disclosure of information to patients in medical care. Medical Care, 1981, 19, 778-783.

Fishbein, M. & Ajzen, A.: Belief, Attitude, Intention, and Behavior: An Introduction to Theory and Research, Reading, Mass.: Addison-Wesley, 1975.

Fishhoff, B.: Cognitive and institutional barriers to "informed consent." In M. Gibson (Ed.), To Breath Freely, Totowa N.J.: Rowan & Allanheld, 1985.

Fishhoff, B.: Judgment and decision making. In R. Sternberg and E. Smith (Eds.) The Psychology of Human Thought, Cambridge University Press: New York, 1986.

Fiske, S.: Schema-triggered affect: Applications to social perception. In M. Clarke & S. Fiske (Eds.) Affect and Cognition: The Seventeenth Annual Carnegie Symposium on Cognition, Hillsdale, N.J.: Erlbaum, 1982.

Folkes, V.: Consumer reactions to product failure: An attributional approach. Journal of Consumer Research, 1984, 10, 398-409.

Gardner, M., Rulien, N., McGhan, W. & Mead, R.: A study of medication information provided by physicians in a health maintenance organization. Drug Intelligence and Clinical Pharmacy, 1988, 22, 596-598.

Gerbert, B.: Perceived likability and competence of simulated patients: Influence on physicians' management plans. Social Science and Medicine, 1984, 18, 1053-1059.

Gerbert, B. & Hargreaves, W.: Measuring physician behavior. Medical Care, 1986, 24, 838-847.

Gilhooley, M.: Learned intermediaries, prescription drugs, and patient information. Saint Louis University Law Journal. 1986, 30, 633-702.

Gillmore, M. & Hill, C.: Reactions to patients who complain of pain: Effects of ambiguous diagnosis. Journal of Applied Social Psychology, 1981, 11, 14-22.

Glenberg, A., Sanocki, T., Epstein, W. & Morris, C.: Enhancing calibration of comprehension. Journal of Experimental Psychology: General, 1987, 116, 119-136.

Green, L., Kreuter, M., Deeds, S. & Partridge, K.: Health Education Planning: A Diagnostic Approach. Mayfield Publishing: Palo Alto, Calif., 1980.

Green, L., Mullen, P. & Friedman, R.: An epidemiological approach to targeting drug information. Patient Education and Counseling, 1986, 8, 255-268.

Greenfield, S., Kaplan, S. & Ware, J.: Expanding patient involvement in care. Annals of Internal Medicine, 1985, 102, 520-528.

Greenwald, A. & Leavitt, C.: Audience involvement with advertising: Four levels. Journal of Consumer Research, 1984, 11, 581-592.

Gutheil, T., Bursztajn, H. & Brodsky, A.: Malpractice prevention through the sharing of uncertainty: Informed consent and the therapeutic alliance. New England Journal of Medicine, 1984, 311, 49-51.

Hall, J. & Dorman, M.: Meta-analysis of satisfaction with medical care: Description of research domain and analysis of overall satisfaction levels. Social Science and Medicine, 1988, 27, 637-644.

Hall, J., Roter, D. & Katz, N.: Task versus socioemotional behavior in physicians. Medical Care. 1987, 25, 399-412.

Hall, J., Roter, D. & Rand, C.: Communication of affect between patient and physician. Journal of Health and Social Behavior, 1981, 22, 18-30.

Hatcher, M., Green, L., Levine, D. & Flagle, C.: Validation of a decision model for triaging hypertensive patients to alternative health education interventions. Social Science and Medicine, 1986, 22, 813-819.

Haynes, B.: A critical review of interventions to improve compliance with special reference to the role of physicians. In M. Knowles (Ed.) Improving Medication Compliance, Washington D.C.: National Pharmaceutical Council, 1985.

Hoch, S. & Deighton, J.: Managing what consumers learn from experience. Journal of Marketing, 1989, 53, 1-20.

Hoff, L.: How often do consumers seek your advice on prescription and OTC drugs? Pharmacy Times, 1975, 163, 52-55.

Holoweiko, M.: Is this the world record for medical malpractice claims? Medical Economics, 1989, 71, 192-211.

Janis, I. & Mann, L.: Decision Making - A Psychological Analysis of Conflict. Free Press: New York, 1977.

Janz, N. & Becker, M.: The health belief model: A decade later. Health Education Quarterly, 1984, 11, 1-47.

Job, S.: Effective and ineffective use of fear in health promotion campaigns. American Journal of Public Health, 1988, 78, 163-167.

Johnson, M.: Comparability and hierarchical processing in multiattribute choice. <u>Journal of Consumer Research</u>, 1988, <u>15</u>, 303-314.

Johnson, W. & Dark, V.: Selective attention. <u>Annual Review of Psychology</u>, 1986, <u>37</u>, 43-75.

Jones, R., Weise, H., Moore, R. & Haley, J.: On the perceived meaning of symptoms. <u>Medical Care</u>, 1981, <u>19</u>, 710-717.

Joyce, C., Caple, G., Mason, M., Reynolds, E. & Mathews, J.: Quantitative study of doctor-patient communication. <u>Quarterly Journal of Medicine</u>, 1969, <u>150</u>, 183-194.

Jugermann, H., Schutz, H. & Thuring, M.: Mental models in risk assessment: Informing people about drugs. <u>Risk Analysis</u>, 1988, <u>8</u>, 147-155.

Kahneman, D. & Tversky, A.: Choices, values, and frames. <u>American Psychologist</u>, 1984, <u>39</u>, 341-350.

Kahneman, D. & Miller, D.: Norm theory: Comparing reality to its alternatives. <u>Psychological Review</u>, 1986, <u>93</u>, 136-153.

Kallen, D. & Stephenson, J.: Perceived physician humanness, patient attitudes, and satisfaction with the pill as a contraceptive. <u>Journal of Health and Social Behavior</u>, 1981, <u>22</u>, 256-267.

Kane, R. & Deuschle, M.: Problems in doctor-patient communications. <u>Medical Care</u>, 1967, <u>5</u>, 260-271.

Kanouse, D., Berry, S., Hayes-Roth, B., Rodgers, W. & Winkler, J.: <u>Informing Patients about Drugs: Summary Report on Alternative Designs for Prescription Drug Leaflets</u>. Santa Monica: Rand Corporation, 1981.

Keown, C., Slovic, P. & Lichtenstein, S.: Attitudes of physicians, pharmacists, and laypersons towards seriousness and need for disclosure of prescription drug side effects. Health Psychology, 1984, 3, 1-11.

Kenny, R.: Between never and always. New England Journal of Medicine, 1981, 304, 1097-1098.

Kindelan, K. & Kent, G.: Patients' preferences for information. Journal of the Royal College of General Practitioners, 1986, 36, 461-463.

Kintsch, W.: The role of knowledge in discourse comprehension: construction-integration model. Psychological Review, 1988, 95, 163-182.

Kiyak, H., Vitaliano, P. & Crinean, J.: Patients' expectations as predictors of orthognathic surgery outcomes. Health Psychology, 1988, 7, 251-268.

Klenenow, D. & Youngs, G.: Changes in doctor/patient communication of terminal prognosis: A selective review and critique. Death Studies, 1987, 11, 263-277.

Klerman, G.: Drugs and social values. The International Journal of the Addictions, 1979, 5, 313-319.

Korsch, B. & Negrete, V.: Doctor-patient communications. Scientific American, 1972, 277, 66-74.

Kraus, N. & Slovic, P.: Taxonomic analysis of perceived risk: Modeling individual and group perceptions with homogeneous hazard domains. Risk Analysis, 1988, 8, 435-455.

Lane, D. & Hutchinson, T.: The notion of "acceptable risk": The role of utility in drug management. Journal of Chronic Diseases. 1987, 40, 621-625.

Lau, R., Bernard, T. & Hartman, K.: Further explorations of common-sense representations of common illnesses. Health Psychology, 1989, 8, 195-219.

Laurent, G. & Kapferer, J.: Measuring consumer involvement profiles, Journal of Marketing Research, 1985, 22, 41-53.

Lee, P. & Lipton, H.: Drugs and the Elderly: A Background Paper. University of California: San Francisco, Ca., 1983.

Leight, K. & Ellis, H.: Emotional mood states, strategies and state-dependency in memory. Journal of Verbal Learning and Verbal Behavior, 1972, 25, 115-120.

Leong, S., Busch, P. & John, D.: Knowledge bases and salesperson effectiveness: A script-theoretic analysis. Journal of Marketing Research, 1989, 26, 164-178.

Leventhal, H.: The role of theory in the study of adherence to treatment and doctor patient-interactions. Medical Care, 1985, 23, 556-563.

Leventhal, H. & Cameron, L.: Behavioral theories and the problem of compliance. Patient Education and Counseling, 1987, 10, 117-138.

Levy, R. Improving patient compliance with medications: Decreasing the total cost of care. In M. Knowles and R. Hurst (Eds.) Pharmaceuticals and Managed Care: Current Issues and Strategies for the '90s. National Pharmaceutical Council: Washington, D.C., 1989.

Ley, P.: Primacy, rated importance, and the recall of medical statements. Journal of Health and Social Behavior, 1972, 13, 311-317.

Ley, P.: Psychological studies of doctor-patient communication. In S. Rachman (Ed.), <u>Contributions to Medical Psychology</u>, New York: Pergamon Press, 1978.

Ley, P. & Morris, L.: The psychology of written information for patients. In S. Rachman (Ed.) <u>Contributions to Medical Psychology</u>, New York: Pergamon Press, 1984.

Linder-Pelz, S.: Social psychological determinants of patient satisfaction: A test of five hypotheses. <u>Social Science and Medicine</u>, 1982, <u>16</u>, 583-589.

Linn, L., DiMatteo, M., Cope, D. & Robbins, A,: Measuring physicians' humanistic attitudes, values, and behavior. <u>Medical Care</u>, 1987, <u>25</u>, 504-513.

Loftus, E.: Informed consent may be hazardous to your health. <u>Science</u>, 1979, <u>204</u>, 11.

Loftus, E. & Fries, J.: Informed consent may be hazardous to your health. <u>Science</u>, 1979, <u>204</u>, 11.

Loftus, E. & Palmer, J.: Reconstruction of automobile destruction: An example of the interaction between language and memory. <u>Journal of Verbal Learning and Verbal Behavior</u>. 1974, <u>13</u>, 585-589.

Maddux, J. & Rogers, R.: Protection motivation and self-efficacy: A revised theory of fear appeals and attitude change. <u>Journal of Experimental Social Psychology</u>, 1983, <u>19</u>, 469-479.

Masson, A. & Rubin, P.: Matching prescription drugs and consumers: The benefits of direct advertising. <u>New England Journal of Medicine</u>, 1985, <u>313</u>, 513-515.

Mayer, J. & Frederiksen, L: Encouraging long-term compliance with breast self-examination: The evaluation of prompting strategies. Journal of Behavioral Medicine, 1986, 9, 179-189.

Mazzuca, S.: Does patient education in chronic disease have therapeutic value? Journal of Chronic Disease, 1982, 35, 521-529.

McCallum, D.: Communicating the Benefits and Risks of Prescription Drugs. Institute for Health Policy Analysis, Georgetown University: Washington, D.C., 1989.

McGuire, W.: The communication-persuasion model and health-risk labeling. In L. Morris, M. Mazis & I. Barofsky (Eds.), Product Labeling and Health Risks, New York: Cold Spring Harbor Laboratory, 1980.

McNeil, B., Pauker, S., Sox, H. & Tversky, A.: On the elicitation of preferences for alternative therapies. New England Journal of Medicine, 1982, 306, 1259-1262.

McNeil, B., Weichselbaum, & Pauker, S.: Fallacy of the five-year survival rate in lung cancer. New England Journal of Medicine, 1977, 299, 1397-1401.

Meyer, D., Leventhal, H. & Gutmann, M.: Common-sense models of illness: The example of hypertension. Health Psychology, 1985, 4, 115-135.

Meyers-Levy, J. & Tybout, A.: Schema congruity as a basis for product evaluation. Journal of Consumer Research, 1989, 16, 39-54.

Mirowsky, J. & Ross, C.: Patient satisfaction and visiting the doctor: A self-regulating system. Social Science and Medicine, 1983, 17, 1353-1361.

Miyake, N. & Norman, D.: To ask a question, one must know enough to know what is not known. Journal of Verbal Learning and Verbal Behavior, 1979, 18, 357-364.

Moore, S., Kalu, M. & Yarvaprabbas, S.: Receipt of prescription drug information by the elderly. Drug Intelligence and Clinical Pharmacy, 1983, 17, 920-923.

Morris, J. & Royle, G.: Offering patients a choice of surgery for early breast cancer: A reduction in anxiety and depression in patients and their husbands. Social Science and Medicine, 1988, 26, 583-588.

Morris, L.: Patient package inserts: A new tool for health education. Public Health Reports, 1977, 92, 421-424.

Morris, L.: The FDA's approach to patient package inserts: The four phases of PPIs. In M. Bogaert, R. Vander Stichele, J. Kaufman & R. Lefebvre (Eds.), Patient Package Insert as a Source of Drug Information, New York: Elsevier Science Publishing Co., 1989.

Morris, L.: Communicating adverse drug effects to patients. Journal of Clinical Research and Development, (in press).

Morris, L.: A marketing perspective on quality of life measurement. In B. Spilker (Ed.), Quality of Life Assessment in Clinical Trials, New York: Raven Press, in press.

Morris, L.: An information processing perspective on doctor-patient communications: Part I: Physician disclosures. Social Pharmacology, 1987, 1, 1-18.

Morris, L.: An information processing perspective on doctor-patient communications: Part II: Patient information processing. Social Pharmacology, 1987, 1, 209-231.

Morris, L., Brinberg, D., Klinberg, R., Rivera, C. & Millstein, L.: Consumer attitudes about advertised medical drugs. Social Science and Medicine, 1986, 22, 629-638.

Morris, L., Brinberg, D., Klinberg, R., Rivera, C. & Millstein, L.: Consumer attitudes about direct advertising of prescription drugs. Public Health Reports, 1986, 101, 82-92.

Morris, L., Brinberg, D. & Plimpton, L.: Prescription drug advertising to consumers: An experiment of source and format, Current Issues and Research in Advertising, 1984, 7, 65-78.

Morris, L. & Groft, S.: Patient package inserts: A research perspective. In D. Melmon (Ed.), Drug Therapeutics: Concepts for Physicians. New York: Elsevier, 1982.

Morris, L., Grossman, R., Barkdoll, G. & Gordon, E.: A segmentational analysis of prescription drug information seeking. Medical Care, 1987, 25, 953-964.

Morris, L. Grossman, R., Barkdoll, G., Gordon, E. & Soviero, C.: A survey of patient sources of prescription drug information. American Journal of Public Health, 1984, 74, 1161-1162.

Morris, L. & Halperin, J.: Effects of written drug information on patient knowledge and behavior: A literature review. American Journal of Public Health, 1979, 69, 47-52.

Morris, L. & Kanouse, D.: Consumer reaction to differing amounts of written drug information. Drug Intelligence and Clinical Pharmacy, 1980, 14, 531-536.

Morris, L. & Kanouse, D.: Informing patients about drug side effects. Journal of Behavioral Medicine, 1982, 5, 363-373.

Morris, L., Mazis, M. & Gordon, E.: A survey of the effects of oral contraceptive patient information. Journal of the American Medical Association, 1977, 238, 2504-2508.

Morris, L. & Millstein, L.: Drug advertising to consumers: Effects of formats for magazine and television advertisements. Food and Drug Cosmetic Law Journal, 1984, 39, 497-503.

Morris, L., Myers, A., Gibbs, P. & Lao, C.: Estrogen PPIs: An FDA survey. American Pharmacy, 1980, 20, 318-322.

Morris, L., Ruffner, M. & Klinberg, R.: Warning disclosures for prescription drugs. Journal of Advertising Research, 1985, 25, 25-32.

Morris, L., Thilman, D. & Myers, A.: Application of the readability concept to patient-oriented drug information. American Journal of Hospital Pharmacy, 1980, 37, 1054-1058.

Morris, L. & Tyson, M.: There is more than one way to go direct to the consumer. Perspectives, 1985, 9, 65-78.

Myers, M., Cairns, J. & Singer, J.: The consent form as a possible cause of side effects. Clinical Pharmacology and Therapeutics, 1987, 42, 250-253.

Nievaard, A.: Communication climate and patient care: Causes and effects of nurses' attitudes to patients. Social Science and Medicine, 1987, 24, 777-784.

Nolan, L. & O'Malley, K.: Prescribing for the elderly: Part I: Sensitivity of the elderly to adverse drug reactions. Journal of the American Geriatrics Society, 1988, 36, 142-149.

Novak, D., Plumer, R., Smith, R., Ochitill, H., Morrow, G. & Bennett, J.: Changes in physicians' attitudes towards telling the cancer patient. Journal of the American Medical Association, 1979, 241, 897-900.

O'Donnell, W.: How much to tell your patient - and when to clam up. Medical Economics, 69, 152-158.

Ortho-Gomer, K., Britton, M. & Rehngvist, N.: Quality of care in an out-patient clinic. Journal of the American Medical Association, 1979, 13, 347-350.

Pascoe, G.: Patient satisfaction in primary health care: A literature review and analysis. Evaluation and Program Planning, 1983, 6, 185-210.

Pauker, S.: Coronary artery surgery: The use of decision analysis. Annals of Internal Medicine. 1976, 85, 8-18.

Pendleton, D. & Bochner, S.: The communication of medical information in general practice consultations as a function of patients' social class. Social Science and Medicine, 1980, 14A, 669-673.

Peguet, B., Wegner, F. & Brown, J.: Prescription drugs: A survey of consumer use, attitudes and behavior. American Association of Retired Persons: Washington, D.C., 1984.

Perri, M.: The direct approach. Pharmaceutical Executive, 1987, 22, 37-42.

Perri, M. & Dickenson, W.: Consumer reaction to a direct-to-consumer prescription drug advertising campaign. Journal of Health Care Marketing, 1988, 8, 66-69.

Petty, R. & Cacioppo, J.: The effects of involvement on responses to argument quantity and quality: Central and peripheral routes to persuasion. Journal of Personality and Social Psychology, 1984, 46, 69-81.

Petty, R., Cacioppo, J. & Schumann, D.: Central and peripheral routes to advertising effectiveness: The moderating role of involvement. Journal of Consumer Research. 1983, 10, 135-146.

Pogge, R.: The toxic placebo: I. Side and toxic effects reported during the administration of placebo medicine. Medical Times, 1963, 91, 773-778.

Pool, J.: Expected and actual knowledge of hospital patients. Patient Counseling and Health Education, 1980, 3, 111-117.

Povar, G., Mantell, M. & Morris, L.: Patients' therapeutic preferences in an ambulatory care setting. American Journal of Public Health, 1984, 74, 1395-1397.

Prather, S.: The choice is yours - communicate or be sued. Medical Economics, 1989, 70, 90-102.

Puto, C.: The framing of buying decisions. Journal of Consumer Research, 1987, 14, 301-315.

Quill, T.: Partnerships in patient care: A contractual approach. Annals of Internal Medicine, 1983, 98, 228-234.

Reidenberg, M. & Lowenthal, D.: Adverse nondrug reactions. New England Journal of Medicine, 1968, 279, 678-679.

Reiser, S.: Words as scalpels: Transmitting evidence in the clinical dialogue. Annals of Internal Medicine, 1980, 92, 837-842.

Rettig, S.: Group discussion and the predicted ethical risk taking. Journal of Personality and Social Psychology, 1966, 3, 629-633.

Rheingold, P.: Products' liability - The ethical drug manufacturer's liability. Rutgers Law Review, 1964, 18, 947, 985-986.

Riley, C.: Patients' understanding of doctors' instructions. Medical Care, 1966, 4, 34-37.

Robinson, E. & Whitfield, M.: Improving the efficiency of patients' comprehension monitoring: A way of increasing patients' participation in general practice consultations. Social Science and Medicine, 1985, 8, 915-919.

Rosenberg, S., Gorman, S., Snitzer, S., Herbst, E. & Lynne, D.: Patients' reaction to physician-patient communication in a mandatory surgical second-opinion program. Medical Care, 1989, 27, 466-477.

Roter, D.: Patient participation in the patient-provider interaction: The effects of patient question asking on quality of interaction, satisfaction, and compliance. Health Education Monographs, 1977, Winter, 281-315.

Roter, D., Hall, J. & Katz, N.: Relations between physicians' behavior and analogue patients' satisfaction, recall, and impressions. Medical Care, 1987, 25, 437-451.

Roter, D., Hall, J. & Katz, N.: Patient-physician communication: A descriptive summary of the literature. Patient Education and Counseling, 1988, 12, 99-119.

Roth, H.: Measurement of compliance. Patient Education and Counseling, 1987, 10, 107-116.

Roth, S. & Cohen, L.: Approach, avoidance, and coping with stress. American Psychologist, 1986, 41, 813-819.

Rothbaum, F., Weisz, J. & Snyder, S.: Changing the world and changing the self: A two-process model of perceived control. Journal of Personality and Social Psychology, 1982, 42, 5-37.

Ruder, Finn & Rotman: Consumer Attitudes Towards Direct Advertising of Prescription Drugs to the Consumer. Ruder, Finn & Rotman: New York, 1985.

Sackett, D. & Haynes, R.: Compliance with Therapeutic Regimens, Baltimore M.D.: Johns Hopkins University Press, 1976.

Safer, M., Tharps, Q., Jackson, T. & Leventhal, H.: Determinants of three stages of delay in seeking care at a medical clinic. Medical Care, 1979, 17, 11-29.

Samora, J., Saunders, L. & Larson, R.: Medical vocabulary knowledge among hospital patients. Journal of Health and Human Behavior, 1961, 2, 83-92.

Sankar, A.: Out of the clinic into the home: Control and patient-physician communications. Social Science and Medicine, 1986, 22, 973-982.

Sauer, F. EEC regulatory initiatives on drug information. In M. Bogaert, R. Vander Stichele, J. Kaufman & R. Lefebvre (Eds.), Patient Package Insert as a Source of Drug Information, New York: Elsevier Science Publishing Co., 1989.

Schwanenflugel, J. & Shoben, J.: Differential context effects in comprehension of abstract and concrete verbal materials. Journal of Experimental Psychology: Learning, Memory and Cognition, 1983, 9, 82-102.

Segall, A. & Roberts, I.: A comparative analysis of physician estimates and levels of medical knowledge among patients. Social Health and Illness, 1980, 2, 317-334.

Shapiro, A., Chassen, J., Morris, L. & Frick, R. Placebo induced side effects. Journal of Operational Psychiatry, 1974, 6, 43-46.

Slovic, P.: Informing and educating the public about risk. Risk Analysis, 1986, 4, 403-415.

Slovic, P., Fischhoff, B. & Lichtenstein, S.: Characterizing perceived risk. In R. Kates, C. Hohenemser & J. Kasperson (Eds.), Perilous progress: Managing the Hazards of Technology, Boulder: Westview, 1985.

Slovic, P., Fischhoff, B. & Lichtenstein, S.: Behavioral decision theory. In. N. Weinstein (Ed.), Taking Care: Understanding and encouraging Self-Protective Behavior. New York: Cambridge University Press, 1986.

Slovic, P., Kraus, N., Letzel, L. & Malmofors, T.: Risk perception of prescription drugs: Report on a survey in Sweden. In B. Horisberger & R. Dinkel (Eds.), The Perception and Management of Drug Safety Risks. New York: Springer-Verlag, 1989.

Smith, C., Polis, E. & Hadac, R.: Characteristics of the initial medical interview associated with patient satisfaction and understanding. Journal of Family Practice, 1981, 12, 283-285.

Smith, J., Falvo, D., McKillip, J. and Pitz, G.: Measuring patient perceptions of the patient-doctor interaction. Evaluation & the Health Professions, 1984, 7, 77-94.

Stafford, L., Burggaf, C. & Sharkey, W.:. Conversational memory: The effects of time, recall, mode, and memory expectations on remembrances of natural conversations. Human Communication Research, 1987, 14, 203-229.

Starfield, B., Steinwachs, D., Morris, I., Bause, G., Siebert, S. & Westin, C.: Presence of observers at patient-practitioner interactions, impact on coordination of care and methodological implications. American Journal of Public Health, 1981, 15, 77-81.

Starfield, B., Wray, C., Hess, K., Gross, R., Birk, P. & D'Lugoff, B.: The influence of patient-practitioner agreement on outcome of care. American Journal of Public Health. 1981, 71, 127-131.

Staudenmayer, M. & Lefkowitz, M.: Direct and indirect measures of patient satisfaction with physician services. Social Science and Medicine, 1981, 15, 77-81.

Stephens, R., Haney, C. & Underwood, S.: Psychoactive drug use and potential misuse among persons aged 55 years and older. In D. Petersen & F. Whittington (Eds.), Drugs, Alcohol and Aging, Dubuque: Kendall/Hunt Publishing Company, 1982.

Stiles, W.: Evaluating medical process components: Null correlations with outcomes may be misleading. Medical Care, 1989, 27, 212-220.

Strull, W., Lo, B. & Charles, G.: Do patients want to participate in medical decision making? Journal of the American Medical Association, 1984, 252, 2990-2994.

Suchman, A. & Mathews, D.: What makes the patient-doctor relationship therapeutic? Connexional dimensions of medical care. Annals of Internal Medicine, 1988, 108, 125-130.

Suls, J. & Fletcher, B.: The relative efficacy of avoidance and nonavoidance coping strategies: A meta-analysis. Health Psychology, 1985, 4, 249-288.

Sujan, M.: Consumer knowledge: Effects on evaluation strategies mediating consumer judgments. Journal of Consumer Research, 1985, 12, 316-321.

Svarstad, B.: Physician-patient communication and patient conformity with medical advice. In D. Mechanic (Ed.), The Growth of Bureaucratic Medicine. New York: John Wiley and Sons, 1976.

Svarstad, B. & Lipton, H.: Informing parents about mental retardation: A study of professional communication and parent acceptance. Social Science and Medicine, 1977, 11, 645-651.

Szasz, T. & Hollander, M.: A contribution to the philosophy of medicine: The basic models of the doctor-patient relationship. Archives of Internal Medicine, 1956, 97, 585-592.

Tabak, E.: Encouraging patient question-asking: A clinical trial. Patient Education and Counseling, 1988, 12, 37-49.

Tabak, E.: The relationship of information exchange during medical visits to patient satisfaction: A review. The Diabetes Educator, 1988, 13, 36-40.

Taylor, K. & Kelner, M.: Interpreting physician participation in randomized clinical trials: The physician questionnaire profile. Journal of Health and Social Behavior, 1987, 28, 389-400.

Taylor, K. & Kelner, M.: Informed consent: The physicians' perspective. Social Science and Medicine, 1987, 24, 135-143.

Taylor, S.: Adjustment to threatening events: A theory of cognitive adaptation. American Psychologist, 1983, 38, 1161-1173.

Thomasma, D.: Beyond medical paternalism and patient autonomy: A model of physician conscience for the patient-physician relationship. Annals of Internal Medicine, 1983, 98, 243-248.

Toogood, J.: What do we usually mean by "usually"? Lancet, 1980, 1, 1094.

Tring, F. & Hayes-Allen, M.: Understanding and misunderstanding of some medical terms. British Journal of Medical Education, 1973, 7, 53-59.

Tuckett, D., Boulton, M. & Olson, C.: A new approach to the measurement of patients' understanding of what they are told in medical consultations. Journal of Health and Social Behavior, 1985, 26, 27-38.

Tversky, A. & Kahneman, D.: The framing of decisions and the psychology of choice. Science, 1981, 211, 453-458.

Tversky, A., Sattah, S. & Slovic, P.: Contingent weighing in judgment and choice. Psychological Review, 1988, 95, 371-384.

Veatch, R.: Voluntary risks to health. Journal of the American Medical Association, 1980, 243, 50-55.

Vertinsky, I., Thompson, W. & Uyeno, D.: Measuring consumer desire for participation in clinical decision making. Health Services Research, 1974, 40, 121-134.

Viscusi, W. & Magat, W.: Learning About Risk: Consumer and Worker Response to Hazard Information. Cambridge: Harvard University Press, 1987.

Wagener, J. & Taylor, S.: What else could I have done? Patients' responses to failed treatment decisions. Health Psychology, 1986, 5, 481-496.

Wallace, L.: Informed consent to elective surgery: The "therapeutic" value? Social Science and Medicine, 1986, 22, 29-33.

Ware, J.: Standards for validating health measures: Definition and content. Journal of Chronic Diseases, 1987, 40, 473-480.

Ware, J. & Hays, R.: Methods for measuring patient satisfaction with specific medical encounters. Medical Care, 1988, 26, 393-402.

Ware, J. & Snyder, M.: Dimensions of patient attitudes regarding doctors and medical care services. Medical Care, 1975, 13, 569-582.

Watenmaker, W. & Shoben, E.: Context and the recallability of concrete and abstract sentences. Journal of Experimental Psychology: Learning, Memory, and Cognition. 1987, 13, 140-150.

Weisman, C., Teitelbaum, M. & Morlock, L.: Malpractice claims experience associated with fertility-control services among young obstetrician-gynecologists. Medical Care, 1988, 26, 298-306.

Weinstein, N.: The precaution adoption process. Health Psychology, 1988, 7, 355-386.

Wertz, D., Sorenson, J. & Heeren, T.: Interpretation of risks provided in genetic counseling. American Journal of Human Genetics, 1985, 39, 253-264.

Wyer, R. & Srull, T.: Human cognition in its social context. Psychological Review, 1986, 93, 322-359.

Yekovich, F. & Walker, C.: Retrieval of scripted concepts. Journal of Memory and Language, 1986, 25, 627-644.

Zaichkowsky, J.: Measuring the involvement construct. Journal of Consumer Research, 1985, 12, 341-352.

Zaichkowsky, J.: Conceptualizing involvement. Journal of Advertising. 1986, 15, 4-14, 34.

Zarin, D. & Pauker, S.: Decision analysis as a basis for medical decision making - The tree of hippocrates. Journal of Medical Philosophy, 1984, 9, 181-213.

Zastoway, T., Roghmann, K. & Hengst, A.: Satisfaction with medical care: Replications and theoretical re-evaluation. Medical Care, 1983, 21, 294-304.